Don Graber M. D.

Gift from
Dr. Coppes at
Seminar at
Southlake Center
for M.H. on
9-27-1997

The Attending Physician

The Attending Physician

Attention Deficit Disorder

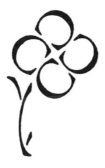

**A Guide for
Pediatricians and
Family Physicians**

Stephen C. Copps, M.D.

Atlanta, Georgia

ISBN 1-880043-02-5
Library of Congress Card Number: 92-082572

Printed in the United States of America

Author

Stephen C. Copps, M.D., is a board-certified pediatrician who has served on the staff of the Gundersen Clinic/La Crosse Lutheran Hospital in La Crosse, Wisconsin since 1961. He is Director of the Comprehensive Child Care Center of the Gundersen Clinic and Director of the Neurodevelopment Evaluation and Treatment Center, Gundersen Clinic/Lutheran Hospital La Crosse. Dr. Copps is also Associate Clinical Professor of Pediatrics, University of Wisconsin, Madison. He received his B.S. degree from the University of Wisconsin and his M.D. from the University of Colorado.

Recognized for his outstanding contributions in pediatric medicine, Dr. Copps has received the American Academy of Pediatrics Award for Outstanding Contribution to the Health Care of Children in Wisconsin, the Arthur L. Turi Award for Outstanding Contribution to Disabled Children, and the Distinguished Alumni Award of the University of Wisconsin's School of Medicine for 1984.

Nationally recognized for his vast experience in the treatment of Attention Deficit Disorder, Dr. Copps lectures widely on the topic.

Dedication

I wish to dedicate this book to the memory of Eric Denhoff, M.D., and David W. Smith, M.D., my mentors at very different times in my life, and my dear friends. I can close my eyes and see them now—both with their open faces, ready smiles and twinkling eyes. I listen, and can again hear those pearls of wisdom issue forth from lips attached to such brilliant minds. Their energy lives on in those of us whose lives they touched so deeply.

Stephen Copps

Acknowledgments

To Bonnie Ritter, our Neurodevelopment Center Coordinator, and to Kalah Haug, her assistant, I am indebted. They typed the manuscript, offered helpful suggestions, corrected my grammar, and injected humor into the task. There should be no sentence that begins with a preposition and nothing left dangling. The encouragement and editing skill of the SPI Press staff are also very much appreciated. Finally, it is most important that I thank the hundreds of parents who have allowed me the privilege of caring for their children. Most of what I know about Attention Deficit Disorder I have learned from them.

Table of Contents

PART II. Diagnosing and Treating
Attention Deficit Disorder

APPENDICES

    DuPaul Rating Scale for ADHA
    Comparison of ADHD/ODD Behaviors (DSM-III-R)
    Comparison of ADHD/ODD/CD Behaviors (DSM-III-R)

Introduction

You are the attending physician. You will have the privilege of attending to the cares and needs of a special group of inquisitive, distractible, busy, maligned youngsters and their troubled, bewildered parents.

These children will challenge your patience and your intellect as they win your hearts. Their mothers and fathers will be eternally grateful to you as you demystify attention deficit disorder and guide them through a myriad of sugary, colored, moldy, allergic, psychogenic misconceptions.

Learn about attention deficit disorder, its diagnosis and treatment, and you will discover the tremendous satisfaction of being the parade marshall for those children who march to the beat of a different drum, never in step. You can do much to shape their lives favorably by preventing secondary disabilities which occur as a result of a life filled with negative consequences for behaviors over which they have little control.

Take on the task. The rewards are great. I dare say that as you perform the necessary first step, that of crawling inside the skin of the ADD child to better understand his feelings and frustrations, you will experience a transformation. If you are intent on bettering the lives of these children, you will never be the same. You may well become a more complete physician.

I would like to have your attention. I will do my best to sustain your interest and keep you focused. I will avoid detailed scientific investigations and psychological jargon. I will keep it simple, factual and practical, while attempting to avoid conflicting prescriptions for action. Attention is the basic neurologic function. Without attention, there can be no education. B. F. Skinner told us that "Education is what survives when what we've learnt has been forgotten." Would that our medical school professors had considered the practicality of that statement.

The ramifications of sustaining focused attention go far beyond the classroom management of the ADD child. The ability to attend has a profound impact on the education of all children. "Give me a child who attends and I can teach the Koran in kindergarten."[1] Too often we overlook the basics. Let's first get the child's attention. When the mind is receptive and focused, the process of education can proceed, often with dramatic results.

If a child has an attention deficit disorder, adaptations and modifications must be made until attention is achieved. Parent and teacher attitudes must be changed; academic demands must be made consistent with the child's learning characteristics; non-compliant behaviors and negative attitudes must be positively addressed; and the neurochemical regulators of attention normalized through medical intervention. These changes can be orchestrated and accomplished by you, The Attending Physician.

♦ ♦ ♦ ♦ ♦ ♦

Attention Is The Basic Neurologic Function.

Without Attention, There Can Be No Education.

PART I

Understanding Attention Deficit Disorder

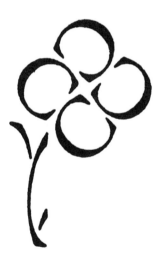

History

In 1845, a family physician, Henrich Hoffman, wrote a book for children entitled *Moral Tales*. Note the word *moral*. That word [moral] helps us to understand some of the guilt parents feel when we talk to them about their children's behavior problems. Hoffman described *fidgety Phil*, the boy who never sat still: "He was a naughty restless child who grew more rude and wild." Obviously the purpose of the book was to warn German children not to be restless and fidgety—characteristics which were not only unappealing but apparently considered immoral as well.

Moral is mentioned again in Dr. George Still's writings. In 1902, he described overly active, disruptive, inattentive children as having "a lack of moral control." Even though Still called the behaviors he observed *a deficit in moral control*, he described a totally new concept, that of biologic morality. He was perhaps the first to attribute this condition to a physiologic cause. His theory was derived from his observations that more often than not such children had responsible, well-intentioned mothers and fathers who did not appear deficient in their parenting skills. For this reason, he eliminated the possibility of a psychogenic cause and attributed the condition instead to a biologic deficit in *inhibitory volition,* a belief consistent with current theory.

During the 1940 encephalitis epidemic, sporadic reports appeared describing children who became disruptive, inattentive, and hyperactive following infectious central nervous system disease. This was called *Brain Damage Behavior Disorder.* By the 1950's, physicians had seen many children with similar symptoms. Most of these children, however, did not appear to have evidence of a physically detectable neurologic deficit. *Minimal Brain Damage,* therefore, became the preferred terminology.

Despite much effort on the part of investigators, no evidence could be found for even minimal brain damage using diagnostic methods available at that time. A school bus carrying children, some diagnosed as having *learning disabilities,* and others diagnosed as having *minimal brain damage,* ran off an icy mountain road in Sweden. Twelve children were killed. Autopsies were performed on six and, by all available technology, including electron microscopy, no brain damage was discernible. Because not even minimal brain damage was detected, and also because the term itself was unpalatable, the name of the condition was once more changed, to *Minimal Brain Dysfunction,* or *MBD.*

As the condition became increasingly thought of as a dysfunction rather than damage, many psychiatrists and psychologists, influenced by the environmental or nurture philosophy of behavioral difficulties, decided, *"If it isn't damage, it must be the result of parental influence."* As a consequence, most professionals forgot Still's suggestion that these characteristics were a result of biologic phenomena. In time, however, it became apparent that medication could alleviate many of the symptoms of the disorder. This response to medication, often quite dramatic, increasingly cast doubt on the psychogenic theory of ineffective parenting.

In the 1970's, the condition was described by its most obvious characteristic, *hyperactivity.* Several years ago, an article, "The Curse of Hyperactivity," appeared in *Time Magazine.* Add a curse to a deficit in moral control and you might consider the need for an exorcist rather than a physician or psychologist. The DSM-II, *Diagnostic and Statistical Manual of Mental Disorders,* published in 1968 by the American Psychiatric Association, referred to the disorder as *Hyperkinetic Reaction of Childhood.* The words *hyperkinesis* and *hyperactivity* are synonymous.

Since many overactive children do not have an attention deficit disorder, the inadvisability of continuing the use of the word hyperactivity as a diagnostic term for the disorder became increasingly apparent. As we entered the 1980's, most professionals in the field began to believe that a deficit in attention was the hallmark of the condition—the core anomaly; hence it came to be known as *Attention Deficit Disorder (ADD)*[2]—a reasonable term and one I shall continue to use, for calling it *Attention Deficit Hyperactivity Disorder*[3] (ADHD) has never made a lot of sense to me. It is also confusing for parents and teachers who have children with attention deficit disorder without hyperactivity.

Attention Deficit Hyperactivity Disorder (ADHD) was the name assigned to this constellation of difficulties in the late 1980's. The definitive symptom is a deficit in attention. The descriptor, *hyperactivity*, fits many children and adolescents with estimates ranging from 60-80%. Others with attention disorders are merely inattentive, distractible and disorganized, while still others are lethargic and process information slowly.

♦ ♦ ♦ ♦ ♦ ♦

ADD BY ANY OTHER NAME IS STILL ADD

- ♦ Lack of moral control.
- ♦ Brain damage behavior disorder.
- ♦ Minimal brain damage.
- ♦ Minimal brain dysfunction (MBD).
- ♦ Hyperkinetic reaction of childhood.
- ♦ Attention deficit disorder (ADD).
- ♦ Attention deficit hyperactivity disorder (ADHD).
- ♦ Who knows what DSM-IV will bring.

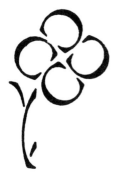

Cause of ADD

Most knowledgeable researchers and practitioners in the field believe that attention deficit disorder is an hereditary developmental disorder which is the result of cerebral neurotransmitter dysfunction. (I would prefer to call it *attention deficit disability* rather than attention deficit disorder.) There is an inherited predisposition for having a child with attention deficit disorder. It is estimated that 30% of fathers and 20% of mothers of children with ADD have residual attention deficit disorder as adults. If one parent has ADD, current estimates suggest a 30% chance of having a child with ADD. If there is an ADD child in the family, there is approximately a 25% chance of occurrence in the next born. Inheritance is polygenic, not autosomal recessive.

Prevalent ADD theory and research suggest that there is a deficiency or imbalance in the catecholamine, dopamine, and perhaps norepinephrine as well, but to a lesser extent. It is not fully understood whether there is a decrease in production or an excessive re-uptake of these cytochemicals. At the present time, it is safe to say there is a wide body of evidence to indicate that this is a biologic dysfunction, but there is no fully accepted biochemical theory. In the past it was suggested that the reticular activating substance in the brain stem was the site of this neurotransmitter dysfunction. It is now believed that a deficiency of transmission of impulses probably affects the entire attention network, including the frontal lobes, the premotor cortex, the limbic system, the basal ganglia, and the reticular activating system, as well as other frontal and central brain structures necessary for attention, inhibition, and motor planning. (Those who would like a more in-depth understanding of the neurophysiology of attention disorders are referred to the references in Appendix A.)

When we later review the characteristics of ADD, you will recognize their close similarity to the behaviors you learned in medical school as those which are associated with frontal lobe damage, behaviors that have to do particularly with inhibition and monitoring. The child with ADD is said by some to have *a deficiency in executive control.* This deficiency results in an inability to maintain or govern selection of goals; in poor anticipation, planning, and carrying out of tasks; and decreased ability to alter plans. Psychological and neuropsychological testing, properly done, can usually distinguish ADD from other cognitive and psychiatric conditions which may produce similar symptoms.

In late fall 1990, an important article appeared in the *New England Journal of Medicine.* The research findings of Alan Zametkin, et al., of the National Institute of Mental Health received acceptance by the scientific community and wide coverage in the lay press. This study showed a definite alteration in glucose metabolism—a decrease in utilization—in certain brain areas of hyperactive adults who were parents of children with attention deficit disorder.[4] This investigation, perhaps more than any other, established ADD as a neurobiological disorder and had a significant impact on the Department of Education's decision to include ADD under the OHI (*Other Health Impaired*) category of Special Education Legislation (Public Law 94-142).

Recently David Comings, reporting in the *Journal of the American Medical Association*, presented convincing evidence for a modifier gene on chromosome 11 common to ADD, Tourette Syndrome and autism. He calls this the *Dopamine D2 receptor locus.*[5]

Many more boys than girls are diagnosed as having the disorder. The ratio of boys to girls with ADD presenting to diagnostic clinics has been reported as being as high as 8:1. It is estimated that the true ratio may be closer to 5:1 or perhaps as low as 3:1. In this manual, I will refer to *him* approximately three times as often as *her*. Perhaps the squeaky wheel gets the grease. Boys with attention deficit disorder are more likely to be diagnosed, for they are often physically more overactive, loud, boisterous and disruptive. Girls, more often than not, do not cause problems. However, they may not perform adequately, especially in school, and may appear withdrawn. The overall incidence of attention deficit disorder is considered to be 3-5% of the school-age population, from preschool through college and some have estimated it to be as high as 7-8%.

The cause of secondary, or acquired, attention deficit disorder, is true brain damage, usually some type of diffuse encephalopathy rather than localized injury. ADD due to brain impairment can generally be separated from primary ADD by a careful history and appropriate physical and laboratory examinations. It is important to stress that there is a true *brain damage behavior disorder*. That designation should not be dropped, for it does apply to some children with the condition. It can occur as a result of lead encephalopathy; infectious central nervous system disease such as encephalitis and meningitis; Rye's Syndrome; hemolytic uremic encephalopathy; elevated bilirubin in sick, immature neonates; fetal alcohol syndrome; and maternal drug usage during pregnancy.

◆ ◆ ◆ ◆ ◆ ◆

CAUSE OF ADD

♦ ADD is a biologic heritable disorder believed to be due to an alteration in neurotransmitter function, mediated by dopamine and perhaps norepinephrine as well.

♦ Many more boys than girls are diagnosed as having ADD.

- The incidence is estimated to be approximately 3 to 5% of the school-age population.

- Acquired ADD is due to brain injury resulting from a variety of cerebral traumas.

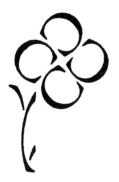

Spurious Causes

True attention deficit disorder is not caused by psychogenic impact on the child. It has a biological cause and is not the result of poor parenting or family dysfunction. It has been said that the child with ADD may create family chaos, but he is not the product of family chaos. The biological cause is not a deficiency in the *maternal hormone*, for too much is usually present. Several years ago, while at the University of Cincinnati, Sylvia Richardson, M.D., stated that she and co-workers had discovered the maternal hormone. This certainly would peak one's interest, for we all know of the fictitious maternal hormone that binds mother to child and results in a myriad of maternal excuses for children's behaviors such as, "She must be tired." Yes, they had discovered the maternal hormone. It is called *guilt*. It is understandable how a mother with a temperamentally difficult, impossible to console, catnapping, up all night, physically overactive infant who resists cuddling, might feel. Failure, depression, anger, frustration, helplessness, and rejection are all common feelings. As the stress continues, she may begin to reject her own infant, and the guilt increases.

Attention deficit disorder is not caused by food additives or preservatives, as Ben Feingold would have had us believe. Nor is it the result of sugar or allergies. Cooperative studies on the effect of food coloring suggest that 2 to 3% of children diagnosed as having attention deficit disorder have a hyperactive response to relatively large amounts of food coloring, the effect appearing within ten minutes of ingestion of the substance and lasting no more than forty-five minutes to one hour. This is strictly an occurrence related in time to the ingestion of the offending substance and in no way causes a persistent pervasive condition.[6] Many physicians witness this phenomenon in their practice when they prescribe very, very orange Erythromycin.

Neither has allergy been found to be a cause of ADD. There is no *brain allergy*. Children who experience allergic symptoms may, as a result of their ill feelings, be inattentive. Antihistamines used in the treatment of allergy can cause drowsiness resulting in off-task behavior. Some children will have an unusual, idiosyncratic hypersensitivity reaction to certain food substances such as soy products, citrus juices, chocolate, etc., which is akin to the reaction to coloring. This hyperkinetic, inattentive reaction is transient and temporally related to the ingestion of the offending agent. There is no evident antigen-antibody reaction and *IGE* is not affected. A hypersensitivity reaction, or true allergy, does not cause the pervasive, persistent condition with discernible characteristics known as *attention deficit disorder*.

Neither is yeast believed to play a significant role.[7,8] It is difficult to take yeast assertions seriously when proponents claim that symptoms of yeast-connected health problems include chronic fatigue, irritability, *PMS*, digestive disorders, muscle pain, short attention span, headache, memory loss, impotence, hyperactivity, depression and learning difficulties, and suggest that psoriasis, multiple sclerosis, chronic hives, autism and arthritis may be yeast connected. (See Appendix N for a position statement from the American Academy of Allergy and Immunology.)

I have great concern when I read such spurious claims. The real danger is that someone might believe them and with-hold appropriate therapy from their children or from themselves.

Sugar is interesting. We are familiar with the markedly variable effect of alcohol, the simplest and most rapidly absorbed sugar. For example, three friends go out for a night on the town; each consumes a considerable amount of whiskey. Tom falls sound asleep; Bill is sick in the bathroom; while Duane is the life of the party as he sings funny, bawdy songs. Three people given alcohol have three different reactions.

Children have similarly unpredictable responses to sugar. I've seen children with attention deficit disorder given a sugar load fall asleep; I've seen others become nauseated; and yet others become increasingly hyperactive. Attention deficit disorder is characterized by exaggerated responses. These exaggerated responses are physiologic as well as behavioral.

There is evidence to suggest that many children with attention deficit disorder, given large quantities of sugar, may experience a transient worsening of their symptoms twenty minutes to a couple of hours after ingestion. They may become overly active if they eat a bowl of sugar-frosted flakes with a tablespoon of sugar and nothing else for breakfast. No one should eat large amounts of refined sugar. It has been suggested by Dr. Keith Conners, a pioneer in ADD, that a more complete breakfast with some protein buffer might protect children with ADD against this sugar effect.[9]

Advice to patients should be characterized by good nutritional sense. All children benefit from a well-balanced diet with required calories, protein, vitamins and minerals. Stress a well-balanced diet and the avoidance of excess to which these children are prone, but don't make a fetish of avoiding sugar, food coloring, or other food-related substances unless there is an obvious indication of an idiosyncratic reaction to an offending agent.

◆ ◆ ◆ ◆ ◆ ◆

SPURIOUS CAUSES

+ Not caused by poor parenting. Guilt fuels the fire.

+ Not the product of family chaos.

+ Not the result of food coloring or preservatives.

+ Not caused by sugar or yeast.

+ There is no *brain allergy.* There can be short-lived, hyperkinetic, hypersensitivity reactions to certain substances——so probably best not to ingest them. Advise a well-balanced, nutritious diet.

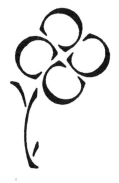

Mimics

Certain conditions may mimic attention deficit disorder. Children with these conditions display some of the characteristics of ADD. Note that I say *some* of the characteristics. When all of the characteristics of ADD are considered, differentiating ADD from the mimics is usually not difficult.

Emotional problems and psychiatric disorders, especially affective or mood disorders, may result in restless, fidgety behavior and inability to concentrate. These disorders generally do not show a persistent, pervasive pattern nor evidence of poor attending since early childhood. When a child has significant anxiety, he may also be restless and fidgety. This condition is characterized by unrealistic worry which is unusual for children with attention deficit disorder, who may show little worry and a notable lack of awareness of the impact of their behavior on others. Because of a faulty feedback loop, the child is not particularly upset with his own actions, for he is unaware he's made a mistake. Although this is true, he is acutely aware of the frustrations experienced by those around him. He is bothered by the negative effects which occur as a consequence of his actions, but he is not aware of his contribution to the negative impact of his behavior. Children with anxiety show symptoms of stress in direct relationship to some event of importance to them, rather than the significant fluctuation in performance, for no apparent reason, so characteristic of children with ADD.

Depression can be present in childhood and true bipolar disorder may be present as well. Depression may result in an inability to concentrate and in inappropriate anger. Depressed persons may blame others (*scapegoating*) or blame themselves, and they are frequently withdrawn and emotionally detached. They may dwell on the past (*gunnysacking*) and often perceive excessive failures of both themselves and others. The child with ADD, by contrast, is more resilient and often does not think about the past. It is common for adolescents and children with attention deficit disorder to have an adjustment reaction with depressed mood rather than true depression. If unrecognized and untreated, the child with ADD may become increasingly anxious and saddened as a result of negative reinforcement and repeated failures.

Characteristics of bipolar disorder that should alert the physician to this possibility include:

1. *Excessive, long-lasting outbursts of anger.* Tantrums that expend tremendous amounts of energy that go on uninterrupted for half an hour to an hour or longer.

2. *Pressured speech.* Children with ADD may talk a lot, but they don't exhibit constant speech for an hour or more, incapable of being interrupted.

3. *Angry destruction.* Children with ADD, because of impulsiveness and hyperactivity, may run into things by accident, but usually do not exhibit vengeful destructiveness.

4. *Sleeping difficulty.* Children with bipolar disorder may get no more than 2-3 hours sleep a night.

5. *Irritability.* Children with ADD do not exhibit the irritability and frequent mood changes common with bipolar disorder.

6.   *Agitation.* The child with ADD is more restless than agitated.

Children with learning disabilities can appear inattentive, fidgety and disruptive as they experience significant frustration in their ability to assimilate academic material. Children, whose ADD-like symptoms are secondary to learning disabilities, do not exhibit the manifestations of the condition prior to being presented with academic material in school. They do well throughout infancy and early childhood without being physically overactive, inattentive or disruptive. Kindergarten goes well unless they are in a so-called *academic kindergarten.* They increasingly have difficulty with attending in first grade in an academic learning situation with which they cannot cope.

On the other hand, ADD can very closely mimic LD. All children considered to be learning disabled should have a thorough ADD evaluation. If ADD is found to be present, it should be treated prior to the establishment of often elaborate and, at times, segregated remedial programs. ADD can impede the acquisition of academic skills. If, after the ADD is appropriately treated, learning disabilities are still evident, they should be remediated and/or appropriate accommodations made.

Atypical absence seizures can result in inattentiveness. Anticonvulsant medication can cause drowsy, inattentive behavior, and often phenobarbital results in a hyperkinetic agitated state, especially in the older child. In fact, it is probably best not to prescribe it as a single anticonvulsant in the child over six.

Auditory processing problems can also be a problem. Often the child staring off into space is having considerable difficulty processing information and appears inattentive because his cerebral computer is working too hard and too slowly.

Deprivation of rejuvenating sleep secondary to sleep apnea results in an inattentive, sluggish child. Sleep apnea is usually caused by enlarged tonsils and adenoids, and is easily corrected.

Though all of the mimics can cause symptoms suggestive of ADD, none results in the complete, recognizable pattern of the disorder.

◆ ◆ ◆ ◆ ◆ ◆

MIMICS

+ Bipolar Disorder—characterized by severe mood swings and irritability. May be overactive at times and depressed at others.

+ Anxiety—characterized by unrealistic worry. The child with ADD is much more carefree.

+ Depression—characterized by dwelling on the past. The child with ADD is typically resilient and is usually positive until the negative effects of failure affect his esteem and sense of well-being.

+ Learning Disabilities—ADD-like behavior appears when the child is presented with academic material he cannot learn.

+ Seizures—loss of contact with environment, postictal lethargic state (epileptiform discharges on sleep-deprived EEG).

+ Auditory Processing Deficits—stares off into space due to processing problems, especially for verbal information.

+ Sleep Apnea—he's tired and inattentive.

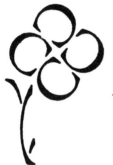

What Is
Attention Deficit Disorder?

The primary characteristics of attention deficit disorder consist of the ADD triad:

> *A deficit in attending ability*—the cerebral regulator is faulty
>
> *Impulsivity*—temperament characteristic of a younger age
>
> *Hyperactivity*—manifest in many but not all youngsters with attention deficit disorder

♦ *A Deficit in Attending*

The problem is not one of attention span. It is evident that youngsters with attention deficit disorder may attend well and for reasonably long periods of time to Saturday morning cartoons on TV, manipulating Micromachines, and to anything that happens to really grab their interest. They will attend if *they* initiate the action, if they are allowed to do so on *their* terms, and if it's something *they* find fascinating. They may even exhibit flypaper attention, which, incidentally, is quite characteristic of the adult with residual attention deficit disorder. Yes, adults may manifest characteristics of attention deficit disorder.

I call it *flypaper attention*. That dates me, but perhaps even the young among you have been told about the sticky roll of flypaper hanging in a coil from the kitchen ceiling. The fly momentarily lights on top of the refrigerator, then zooms in his hyperactive manner across the room to the stove, immediately leaves the stove, and lands on a light fixture. As he lands, he eyes the banana peel left on the counter. On his way to the peel, he is distracted by the sweet smell of flypaper and whammo! he's stuck and cannot be dislodged. When the person with ADD gets stuck on something in which he is interested, nothing may be able to dislodge him from the task. This characteristic is sometimes referred to as being *overfocused* and may contribute to his inflexibility. Once he's made up his mind, that's the way it's going to be.

The problem with attention appears to be one of regulation. Children with ADD usually can initiate attention, but they have considerable difficulty sustaining attention. It has been said, "They are good starters but poor finishers; they are quick out of the gate, but fade in the stretch."

Children with ADD may have difficulty focusing their attention on the most appropriate subject. They have difficulty selecting from a variety of stimuli the one to which they should be attending. As a classroom teacher said, "They attend to everything but what they're supposed to be paying attention to." It is often the teacher's voice they ignore. Their regulator of attention is faulty.

♦ *Impulsivity*

Impulsivity is characteristic of the two-year-old. One mother said to me, "My child, now 14, entered the 'terrible two's' and never left." The child with ADD is impulsive. He cannot delay gratification. He requires immediate, repetitive, intrinsic gratification. He has little regard for yesterday, and tomorrow is equally meaningless. *Right now is where it's at.* He learns from what is going on about him at the moment, not from what people tell him and especially not from those far-off rewards promised him. This is why report cards four weeks or even two weeks ahead have little meaning. A more effective reward is an ice cream cone right now rather than a trip to the zoo next weekend.

Cognitively, ADD children know what to do. They know they should think before they act, but they don't do it. Attempting to teach them skills, whether social skills or attending skills, may hold little meaning. They are managed primarily by immediate consequences. They're too impulsive to be governed effectively by rules such as "don't interrupt." They know not to interrupt; they just can't do it. As a precious first-grade girl sadly reported, "I always lose my crayons (the negative reward system) for talking. I don't mean to; I just forget." The impulsive nature of the ADD child accounts for the failure of many behavior management programs which assume the child will think before acting.

♦ *Hyperactivity*

The word means nothing more than increased physical activity. How many times we've said,'"Oh, if I could only have some of his energy!" All children who are hyperactive do not have attention deficit disorder. Some have extraordinary selective attention and are not the least bit distractible. In 1982, I gave a talk at a meeting of the American Academy of Pediatrics: "A Pediatrician Looks at Hyperkinesis." I reviewed for the audience the differential diagnosis of hyperactivity and talked about the hyperactive youngster with excellent attending ability. He leaves point "A" and travels in his hyperactive manner to point "B". On the way he is asked a question. He lights at point "B" and gives the answer. He studies with the stereo blaring, the dog barking and his siblings fighting. He has marvelous selective attention and is constantly on the go. I referred to that youngster as the *Datsun child*, for Datsun Motor Company at that time had a slogan, "We are driven." The Datsun child does not have attention deficit disorder, but hyperactive he is!

Some children who exhibit hyperactivity may have a *bipolar disorder* (formerly manic-depressive illness). If this overly active child has severe mood swings and is frequently irritable, or if there is a family history of bipolar disorder or depression, be sensitive to this possibility, especially if he exhibits the bipolar characteristics listed in the section entitled *Mimics*.

Some children with ADD are not hyperactive— they're just not. We do not know why this is any more than we know why some children with Down's Syndrome don't have slanted eyes—they just don't. Not being hyperactive may be related to the sedentary habits of the parents, the child being normally active, but hyperactive in comparison with the parents' kinesthetics. The obese child with ADD is less likely to be obviously hyperactive and, in general, girls appear to be less hyperactive than boys, though some now dispute that suggestion.

Some children who appear to have ADD without hyper-activity have significant visual and/or auditory processing deficits. Their spaciness may be related to processing difficulty rather than true ADD. On the other hand, there are those who appear to have auditory processing deficits who, in fact, have ADD. Those children are markedly distracted by light and movement, as well as sound.

It has been suggested that perhaps many children with ADD symptoms, who are not hyperactive, are inattentive due to anxiety.[10] This theory may explain why children with apparent ADD without hyperactivity are more apt to exhibit affective disorders. Children with ADD with hyperactivity, especially if properly treated, are unlikely to experience clinical anxiety or depression.

An occasional child will appear inattentive and underactive (hypoactive) on the basis of hypothyroidism. Order a T-4 and sensitive TSH (STSH). Weigh more heavily the TSH in determining the child's metabolic state. Beyond infancy, use that parameter to follow thyroid replacement therapy. Some with an attention deficit and normal thyroid function are lethargic and withdrawn—especially girls.

◆ ◆ ◆ ◆ ◆ ◆

ATTENTION DEFICIT DISORDER IS . . .

+ A deficit in the regulation of attention.

+ Impulsivity as it relates to immediate, intrinsic gratification.

+ Hyperactivity in most.

ALL ARE NOT HYPERACTIVE

+ Some are not hyperactive—they're just not.

+ Some are not hyperactive—they have an ADD look-a-like due to processing deficits.

+ Some are not hyperactive—they have an ADD look-a-like due to anxiety.

+ Some are hypoactive—suspect hypothyroidism.

+ Some have an attention deficit with lethargic, withdrawn behavior—especially girls.

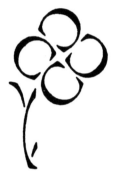

New Light

New Light—perhaps, or likely, or even probable, but let's be careful not to become blinded by that light.

Russell Barkley, Ph.D., whom I consider one of the foremost researchers in ADD, has suggested that the culprit in ADD is not a deficit in attention but a lack of motivation.[11] "Russ," I want to say, "how could you?" It has taken us so long to have ADD recognized as an entity. As confusing and imprecise as the term may be, it has gained wide acceptance and is not nearly as misunderstood as the term *motivational deficit*.

I'm going to tell you what I think Dr. Barkley means while doing my best to preserve attention deficit disorder (ADD) as an acceptable name for this complicated condition. I feel it's important that this be done, for we have worked hard to finally convince teachers that the inattentive children in their classes may well have a biologic deficit in the regulation of attention and are not just poorly motivated, or *lazy*, as many have suggested.

Dr. Barkley's word *motivation* does not refer to the Vince Lombardi, Dale Carnegie, pull-yourself-up-by-your-own-bootstraps type of motivation we all associate with the word. He refers to that as *cognitive motivation*. That is not what he means when he talks of the ADD child as having a motivational deficit. He, being the good scientist he is, is seeking the behavioral characteristic most common to the condition —that which serves to explain all of the characteristics. He is striving to discern the common root. When he uses the word *motivation*, he is talking science, not football, scholarship or business success.

The motivation to which he refers is *motivation by consequence* which he theorizes is lacking in ADD. Some have called this a lack of incentive motivation. He asserts that ADD is caused by a biologic cerebral deficit which numbs the child's sensitivity to consequences and rules. It is his impression that these children have a deficit in how behavior is managed by rules, a deficit in *rule-governed behavior*. This is not unlike George Still's impression back in the early 1900's when he spoke of a biologic deficit in *inhibitory volition*.

This theory, which is becoming widely accepted, has tremendous implications for the management of ADD. This is important, for basing management on attempts to improve attention in traditional ways has not been especially beneficial. Cognitively, these children know what to do, they simply cannot do it. Reasoning and explanation are notably ineffective. The rewards and punishments which change the behaviors of others do not seem to work for the child with ADD. Rather, the magnitude of both must be increased and additional cognitive cueing strategies employed to catch the attention of the child with ADD and to promote change.

I would hope that we could all come to understand what Dr. Barkley means by *motivational deficit*, then avoid using the word in reference to ADD in polite company. Let's avoid using the word for the same reason we avoid using the term *hypo-arousal* in referring to the ADD child. We avoid using hypo-arousal because it is misunderstood. There may well be a biologic hypo-arousal related to dopamine deficiency resulting in poor regulation of ADD behaviors, but if you ever told a parent or teacher that their *Jumpin' Johnny*[12] was underaroused, they would think you had taken leave of your senses.

Motivation, as a term to describe an insensitivity to consequences, will be misunderstood. It may well be the behavioral root problem, but the results are the same. ADD children are inattentive (much of the time), are impulsive (most of the time), and the majority are hyperactive (when they shouldn't be). Attention, impulsivity and hyperactivity are tangible occurrences we can observe. Many will have a hard time understanding consequential or incentive motivation. This concept is probably too confusing for most parents and teachers, and these are the persons we must reach.

As we attempt to illuminate behavioral etiology, let's not allow common sense to evaporate as science takes over. As G. K. Chesterton so aptly phrased it, let's not "throw out the baby with the bath water."

♦ ♦ ♦ ♦ ♦ ♦

NEW LIGHT

♦ It has been suggested that the behavioral etiology is a biologic deficit in motivation, not attention.

♦ It is not cognitive, Vince Lombardi-type motivation, but a deficit in being motivated by consequences.

♦ ADD may be considered to be a deficit in being motivated by rules—a problem in rule-governed behavior.

♦ Let's not change the name of the disorder. Let's call it ADD. Attention, impulsivity and hyperactivity are tangible occurrences we can all observe and understand.

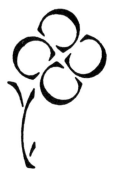

DSM-III-R Criteria
for Diagnosis

There are fourteen behaviors listed in the DSM-III-R as being characteristic of attention deficit hyperactivity disorder.[3] They appear in descending order of discriminating power. To consider the diagnosis, these behaviors must be present to a greater extent than that considered usual for a person of a given mental age. These symptoms must have been present for over six months and have made their appearance prior to age seven. The child with attention deficit disorder with hyperactivity should exhibit at least 8 of the 14.

> 1. *Often fidgets.* I heard a school psychologist refer to this as the *squirm count.* Children with attention disorders are restless and fidgety . . . and the longer they must sit quietly or the less interesting the task for them, the more restless they become.

---

2. *Difficulty remaining seated.* This characteristic of the ADD child is very typical in the
early grades. As he gets older, he may stay in
his chair, but other parts of his body move,
especially his lips.

3. *Easily distracted.* I have often used Mel
Levine's example of three children sitting in
a school classroom. A fire engine goes by a
block away. The first child doesn't even look
up; the second momentarily lifts his head
from his paper, then returns to his
arithmetic; while the third is distracted from
task for several minutes wondering how
many fire engines went to the fire, was an
ambulance there, how much damage was
done and was anyone hurt. That is the
youngster who may well have an attention
deficit disorder.

4. *Difficulty awaiting his turn.* What he has to
say is so important it must be said now.
Waiting in a line is next to impossible.

5. *Often blurts out answers to questions.* How
familiar school teachers are with this
particular incompetent behavior. I think we
should use the term *blurt ratio*, that is, the
ratio between the number of times the child
raises his hand and is called upon compared
to the number of times he blurts out the
answer or offers advice. Most first-grade
teachers can identify a child with an
attention deficit disorder and they are
frequently right. They use the squirm count
and the blurt ratio, which, when used in
combination, are often good predictors of
ADD.

6. *Difficulty following through on instructions.*
She may initiate appropriate action, but may
soon forget what she's to do, become
distracted by a more interesting stimulus, or
lose interest.

7. *Difficulty sustaining attention.* Fades in the stretch—soon becomes bored—can't sustain the effort.

8. *Shifts from one uncompleted task to another.* If repetitive encouragement isn't there to keep him focused, the novelty of a new stimulus will capture his attention. He doesn't purposely wander; rather, novelty is stimulating and he is constantly alert to it, rather than the more familiar task at hand.

9. *Difficulty playing quietly.* This is true except when engrossed in legos or taking apart the radio. I've learned from my patients that there is a marvelous construction toy great for ADD kids and their preference for kinesthetic learning. It's called *Capsela®* and comes complete with a motor, precision-fitted gears, drive trains, and the potential for intense absorption and the creation of amazing moving vehicles.[13]

10. *Often talks excessively.* May be quiet for relatively long periods of time when engrossed in a novel task, but in interpersonal relations is impulsive and often talks non-stop. This is not the constant pathological, pressured speech seen in bipolar disorder.

11. *Often interrupts.* Particularly when mother is on the phone. For some reason, the telephone acts as a magnet. As soon as it rings and Mom starts talking, the child is compelled to talk to her. Interestingly enough, adults with residual ADD often manifest this same behavior.

12. *Does not seem to listen.* This is characteristic of many children with primary ADD. It might also be a mimic. Some children have a deficit in processing auditory information.

The teacher may say, "I don't think the child can hear." A hearing test is performed which reveals normal hearing. The teacher still doesn't think the child can hear. Results of another hearing test return perfectly normal. A month later the teacher is still convinced the child can't hear, but unfortunately, by this time, she has given up or is beginning to think it might be her imagination. This scenario is characteristic of the youngster who is having difficulty processing auditory information. These children also appear to be distractible but, unlike the child with attention deficit disorder, the child is distracted by extraneous noise and not by other stimuli, such as light or motion. There is a significant overlap in ADD and auditory processing dysfunction. Thus, differential diagnosis is critical.

13. *Often loses things.* This is especially true of homework assignments and notes to be taken home regarding the PTA bake sale ... or a conduct slip. Impulsivity and disorganization result in messy rooms, desks and lockers in which wanted objects disappear.

14. *Engages in physically dangerous activities.* The ADD child acts on impulse without considering consequences. Many also seek high levels of sensory stimulation which result in high-risk behaviors. It might be advisable to discourage three-wheelers and motorcycles. Driving, without medication and previous behavior management and responsibility programs, can also be a dangerous activity for teens with ADD.

Please consider this constellation of characteristics a screening tool, not a diagnostic instrument. Your clinical judgment, in conjunction with these markers, is crucial.

I find that having 8 of the 14 characteristics is not reliable enough for the younger child. I require 10 of 14 to be present in the child three to six years of age, 8 for the child six to twelve, and 6 of the 14 for the child twelve to eighteen years of age. As the child matures, he often demonstrates fewer characteristics of the disorder. Perhaps his frontal-lobe monitoring, executive-function/ feedback loop is maturing. This has given rise to the erroneous impression that ADD is outgrown. I feel that the condition should be manifest before four years of age, not seven, and be present for at least one year, not six months.

I choose not to make the diagnosis in a child under three years of age, for so many ADD behaviors are characteristic of two-year-old performance. I consider some children to be at risk for developing attention deficit disorder even when they are one year of age or younger. They are temperamentally difficult children. Mothers must understand, with your help, that these temperamentally difficult children with erratic sleeping habits who seem always discontent, and who are unresponsive to touch and holding, are not banging into things and disrupting family life because of something parents are doing wrong. These children are difficult temperamentally and should be considered to be at risk for developing ADD.

It is estimated that approximately one-third to one-half of these children, who are temperamentally difficult at two years of age, will be shown to have ADD. Genetic influence not only shapes body build and physical appearance but one's temperament as well. ADD is a temperamental variant and, if severe enough, a disability.

♦ ♦ ♦ ♦ ♦ ♦

DSM-III-R CHARACTERISTICS OF ADD[3]

- Fidgety
- Difficulty remaining seated
- Easily distracted
- Difficulty waiting
- Often blurts out (at inappropriate times)
- Difficulty following through on instructions
- Difficulty sustaining attention
- Shifts from one uncompleted task to another
- Difficulty playing quietly
- Talks excessively (when the subject interests him)
- Interrupts
- Does not seem to listen
- Loses things
- Engages in physically dangerous activities

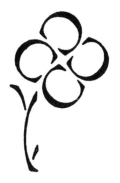

Other Characteristics
of ADD

Over the years I have developed a list of characteristics which I find of considerable help in making a correct diagnosis and separating attention deficit disorder from other conditions.

Many children with attention deficit disorder have an *extraordinary memory for remote events*, especially when compared with their short-term memory. I have often heard a mother comment on this ability, shake her head and say, "I just can't believe the things that child remembers from years ago." This is confusing, for the ADD child may be unable to remember what he has just been told. What he remembers from the distant past relates to his experiences, not to math facts or history dates. These children remember life, not bits of information.

Extraordinary attention to detail. Many children with ADD reveal extraordinary attention to detail, especially if creative and more visual in their learning style. I have seen ADD youngsters draw eighteen wheels on a tank, a whole army of ants, the stitches in shirts, and individual bricks in the wall.   There often is extraordinary attention to detail in their drawings.   This same child may be unable to pick out the hidden figures in *Highlights Magazine*.   These children often have a difficult time with figure-ground perception represented by embedded-figure tasks. Attention to detail may also include attention to the minutest detail of their surroundings.   On the other hand, some ADD children appear unaware of details.

They take it all in. I call them *human wide-angle lenses*. A lens takes little pieces of light and brings them together to a central point for our recognition.   Many of these children walk into a room and are immediately aware of every picture on the wall, what you are wearing, who is frowning, who is smiling, and the color of the kitty cat.

There is *marked fluctuation in performance* without apparent reason.   This helps significantly in differentiating ADD from other conditions such as anxiety and depression.   There is variation in both behavior and academic performance, not only from day to day, but sometimes from hour to hour. They generally do better in the morning than in the afternoon, for as the day goes on they become increasingly bored.   Many a mother with a child with ADD will tell you her child will go from being a devil to an angel and back again in a matter of minutes. ADD children appear to be both inconsistent and unpredictable.   Most, however, are sensitive and caring underneath their seeming obliviousness.

I've always considered this marked fluctuation in perform-ance to be without cause, but now I'm not so sure.   Much of it may be related to whether or not the child is receiving immediate intrinsic gratification at the time.   If there is a goodness of psychological fit between the child, complete with his deficits, and his present environment, ADD symptoms may not be manifest.

This fluctuation in behavior, which is perhaps one of the most dramatic and confusing characteristics of ADD, partially explains why some scientists have dropped the attention model and are seeking other explanations.   Theories include a deficit in sustaining effort, a deficit in rule-governed behavior, and a deficit in the ability to be guided by consequences. If it were just a deficit in attention, the inattentiveness should always be present, and it is not.

Often children with ADD have *difficulty internalizing the rules.* Others know the rules, but impulsively break them. Thus, when an effective plan of management is developed, it must continue or the child will return to the original behavior. This child will not carry out your bidding when you leave the room, for he has lost your effect as governor of his behavior. His own faulty governor is not up to the task. Consistent behavior management programs, especially when combined with positive cognitive-cueing, may, over time, result in new patterns of behavior.

Flight of ideas is another trait. The child's train of thought is sometimes fascinating and is usually imaginative, but it is difficult to follow the story line. One child with ADD described a visit to her grandmother in this way: "Pigeons fly a long way to get home. I flew to grandma's. She's in Florida. I liked looking at the clouds, but Disney World was better. Grandma's better. She was sick. Planes crash—ours didn't. How do those birds know where home is?" Her train of thought doesn't stay on the track, for the child has too much difficulty organizing. She can't attend to what she just said in order to connect it to what she is about to say. Irrelevant thoughts are often not inhibited but may be added to the story line. Such divergent thinking can be creative, but more often is confusing to the listener and disruptive of the child's logical and sequential thought processes.

It is important to recognize that the child can be *internally distracted as well as externally distracted.* She may be distracted by her growling stomach. He may be distracted by a tight belt, a pebble in his shoe, or a little bit of fantasy. It is understandable that a youngster who has experienced a great deal of negativism may occasionally retreat into a little dream world in which he is king. Fantasizing oneself as Darth Vader may be much more enjoyable than struggling with geography. Fantasy and internal distractions may account for his not getting his work done even when he is in an isolation cubicle.

The child with attention deficit disorder *requires instant gratification.* Remote rewards are relatively meaningless to him. He needs to know what's in it for him *now* and he has to hear it over and over again. Incidentally, adults with residual ADD have these same characteristics. Dad just finishes adding a new handle to the door latch and yells out to his wife, "Hey, honey, come see this. It works like a charm, better than new, I knew I could do it myself. What do you think of that? You do think it's good, don't you? Do you really like it?"

Many persons with ADD are emotionally volatile. *They may overreact* to anything, from minor illness to injury. There is *marked intensity.* There is electricity in the air, particularly when they are on a roll. The adult with attention deficit disorder often exhibits this same characteristic. When he is interested in something, he may come on pretty strong. He often exhibits considerable intensity, of which he is unaware. This intensity may result in rejection by his audience, be it his wife or a colleague at work.

Many children with ADD have a *lack of respect for boundaries.* There is lots of physical touching and contact. Witness the mother in the kitchen with the child constantly tugging at her skirt. The older ADD child or adult may inadvertently tug or touch, hug or slap on the back to the consternation of the recipient. This lack of sensitivity to boundaries can lead to rejection as early as kindergarten by children whose needs for interpersonal space must be respected. The problem may continue for a lifetime.

Poor organizational skills. Inability to organize oneself, one's belongings, time requirements, etc., is a major problem for most children, adolescents and adults with ADD. In fact, ADD in adults has been called *Adult Disorganization Disorder.* Poor organizational skills are a major problem for the ADD child at school. Just take a look at their school desks. Often it is not that ADD children have not completed their daily work, which is also pretty characteristic, but rather they cannot find it amid the crumpled papers, rubber bands, pieces of broken pencils, legos and half of last week's sandwich.

Failure to anticipate consequences. It is important to realize that youngsters with attention deficit disorder usually do not appreciate the consequences of their actions and fail to think ahead about consequences before they act. They often feel that it is the rest of the world that has the problem. This is very different from scapegoating or blaming others. The blaming of others can be oppositional or it may be associated with depression.

Great difficulty with transitions. Most ADD children like things just the way they *were.* This is characteristic of the adult with residual attention deficit disorder as well when he says, "Why did you move that picture?" or the one who is distressed when his chair has been moved to the other side of the window, especially if the magazine rack is no longer on the left. There may be difficulty in transition from one room to another in school, or from one teacher to another, as occurs in middle and high school. Transition may be especially difficult when returning from an unstructured to a structured setting, such as coming in from recess. This difficulty with transitions relates to the child's sense of disorganization.

The child with ADD *complains of boredom.* The most typical utterance is, "I'm bored." This may be the tipoff that she is having difficulty accomplishing her work, whatever it might be. Take a hard look at the demands placed upon the child and what might be disturbing the goodness of fit. Often it is not enough feedback. It may also reflect a lack of adequate stimulation from the tasks. Or, he may be overwhelmed by the demands and shut down, rationalizing that he is bored when, in reality, he cannot do the task.

The child, adolescent and adult with ADD is apt to be *brutally frank* or unnecessarily candid. The parent or spouse is often embarrassed by the outspoken nature of appraisal or the detailed description of dislike.

Fatigue is common. You might say, "What do you mean fatigue is common? These kids are atomic-powered. They are indefatigable." Yes, indeed, they are, but when they crash, they crash. They either go out like a light or, after an extended period of extreme activity if they're not in a place where they can crash, they just barely drag themselves about.

In infancy they may have *erratic sleeping habits*, often catnapping. They rarely give mom a chance to get her work done, for it seems that as soon as they fall asleep, they are up banging on the sides of their crib. Later in childhood, when every other three-year-old is taking a nap, they have no interest in sleeping at all. In kindergarten they won't stay on the mat. They are generally *restless sleepers* and may experience *night terrors*, but usually awaken refreshed and raring to go. They have night terrors which do not interrupt sleep, as opposed to nightmares which awaken the child.

An adult with attention deficit disorder should be aware that, as he closes his eyes and falls asleep, he may lose some of his charm. He may thrash and turn, flail his arms about, butt his wife in the fanny, grab a corner of the blanket and curl up like a cocoon.

He often doesn't just talk in his sleep, he may yell or even scream. He awakens refreshed, and looks down at his wife lying on the cold floor in her nightgown. "Sleep well, honey?" He then bounds off to the bathroom leaving the door wide open as he uses the toilet. When he approaches the sink to shave, he remembers his wife said something about the toilet seat. He can't remember whether she said to put it up or down, so he flips it up. Ten minutes later when she comes into the bathroom, she falls through and he wonders why he tries her patience.

Kinesthetic learning is generally not affected by ADD. How often these children say, "Don't tell me, show me." This is why motor manipulative toys are so enjoyed and are so beneficial to the ADD child. It is critical that multisensory approaches which include visual, auditory, tactile and kinesthetic modalities be utilized in their education.

OTHER CHARACTERISTICS OF ADD

- Remarkable memory for experiences in the distant past
- Extraordinary attention to detail
- Keen ability to take it all in
- Marked fluctuation in performance
- Flight of ideas
- Internally as well as externally distracted
- Instant gratification required
- Marked intensity
- Little respect for boundaries
- Poor organizational skills
- Failure to anticipate consequences
- Difficulty with transitions
- Boredom
- Fatigue
- Erratic sleeping habits
- Difficulty internalizing

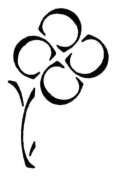

The Modifiers

Certain conditions will modify attention deficit disorder. When these modifiers are present, the characteristics of the disorder may disappear. The child will not generally appear distracted or hyperactive when things are interesting or if it is a first-time, *novel* experience. *Intimidation* can momentarily control symptoms of attention deficit disorder. Many of the manifestations will disappear in a *one-on-one* situation in a *quiet* environment. Their governor is close to them and there are few distractions. These modifiers are the reason it is difficult to diagnose ADD from observations of behavior in the school psychologist's office or in the pediatrician's examining room. Escort Johnnie to the testing area. It may be intimidating, for he's never been there before. The one-on-one attention from an Examiner focuses his attention. Give him a test he's never seen. It's interesting dealing with all those different shapes. It is also a new situation. The great majority of children with attention deficit disorder will show few, if any, of the characteristics of the disorder under these conditions.

There may be no observable attention deficit symptoms when the child is receiving *persistent repetitive feedback*. This is the reason these children require constant encouragement in the classroom. It also explains why Nintendo is their passion, while a book report is their nemesis. Illness, too, sometimes overshadows the ADD. A sick child may not have the energy to be overactive or impulsive.

♦ ♦ ♦ ♦ ♦ ♦

THE MODIFIERS

Many characteristics of ADD disappear
when there is:

♦ Intimidation

♦ A new or novel experience

♦ A one-on-one situation

♦ A quiet environment

♦ Something of interest

♦ Constant repetitive feedback

♦ Illness

The Co-Morbidities

In caring for youngsters with attention deficit disorder, we should be aware of conditions which may be associated with ADD but are not part of the disorder. These are the *co-morbidities*, the commonest of which is oppositional defiant (noncompliant) behavior disorder, or ODD. In my own practice no more than 35% of the youngsters I see with ADD have an oppositional behavior disorder. Oppositional defiant behavior may be unrelated to the attention deficit disorder. It may exist as a consequence of family disruption or dysfunction. On the other hand, it may be secondary to attention deficit disorder as a consequence of years of negative reinforcement.

A conduct disorder (CD) may co-occur with attention deficit disorder. Conduct disorders are characterized by setting fires, stealing outside the home, assault and battery, prolonged truancy, smoking at a young age and sexual abuse. Drinking alcohol in childhood is often included in conduct disorder, while alcoholism, because of its addictive nature, should be in a separate category.

Some children with or without attention deficit disorder show severe aggressive behavior. I do not like to see this, particularly in young children. It is a poor prognostic sign, especially when it involves physical abuse of other people or animals. Such children must be treated very early and vigorously, for long-term prognosis is quite poor. Often the significantly aggressive preschooler is experiencing attachment anxiety and fears rejection. Despite this, he seems to do everything in his power to see to it that his fear is justified. These children are at risk for severe antisocial behavior as they get older. Aggressive children require much positive interaction and much behavioral intervention to, hopefully, attain social competency. All too often the severity of this problem is underestimated and, as a result, is undertreated.[14]

Many children with attention deficit disorder have concomitant learning disabilities. It is estimated that approximately 30% of youngsters with ADD have specific learning disabilities (SLD), and that 75% will be at least one grade level behind in at least one subject by third grade. It appears that language-based learning problems are more common than difficulty with mathematics, at least at the conceptual level. Children with ADD often experience difficulty with temporal sequential organization, short-term memory and word retrieval or *nominal aphasia*, an inability to come up with the right word at will. In testing for temporal sequential organization, it is interesting to see how many can rapidly recite the days of the week or the months of the year but cannot tell you what comes after Thursday or before September.

Anxiety and true depression may co-occur with ADD. They may also mimic ADD in that they have characteristics in common with attention deficit disorder. Sometimes in the very young or older child, differentiation is difficult.

♦ ♦ ♦ ♦ ♦ ♦

CO-MORBIDITIES

♦   Oppositional defiant behavior disorder (ODD).

♦   Conduct disorder (CD).

♦   Learning disabilities (LD).

♦   Aggressive behavior.

♦   Anxiety and depression can mimic ADD and also co-occur with it.

Incompetent ADD Behavior vs. Noncompliance

It is imperative in our understanding of attention deficit disorder that we become aware of the difference between the incompetent, sometimes called *skill-deficit*, behaviors that occur as a consequence of attention deficit disorder and noncompliant, oppositional defiant behaviors. The DSM-III-R has done a commendable job in differentiating the behaviors which characterize the different disorders.

Attention deficit disorder is a developmental disability which is the result of a neurobiologic disturbance. We should no more punish the child with attention deficit disorder for his incompetent behaviors than we should chastise a youngster with cerebral palsy because he limps. Behaviors listed under attention deficit disorder should be regarded as characteristic of the condition. The child should not be punished when they occur. Parents and teachers must become governors or regulators of these behaviors. While they should not be punitive, neither should they let inappropriate, incompetent behavior go unattended without comment, such as "Please don't interrupt, I'm talking to your father." Oppositional, noncompliant behaviors, on the other hand, must be recognized as such and dealt with through specific behavioral interventions which may include both positive and negative consequences.

I suggest you make copies of the DSM-III-R sheet in Appendix E, for you will find it useful in helping parents understand the important distinction between the behaviors typical of each disorder. It can be anticipated that medication will have a beneficial effect on reducing those behaviors resulting from ADD. On the other hand, it is important to stress to teachers, as well as to parents, that little significant improvement in noncompliant behaviors as a result of medication should be anticipated. The child must be held accountable for opposition and defiance, and disciplined accordingly. These behavior problems must be dealt with behaviorally.

Too often, oppositional, defiant behaviors have been confused with behaviors caused by ADD. They have been included as characteristic of ADD, and they are not. This is one of the reasons that outcome research has been fraught with so much inaccuracy and inconsistency.

The presence of conduct disorder must also be assessed. I've included another sheet in Appendix E which lists the characteristics of all three behavior disorders side by side. I made two separate sheets, for I use the one listing the characteristics of conduct disorder sparingly. I find it of some value in helping persons understand where the child might be headed without appropriate intervention.

◆ ◆ ◆ ◆ ◆ ◆

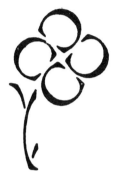

Desirable Traits

Lest we become too engrossed in incompetent and noncompliant behaviors, consider for a moment the desirable traits of most children with attention deficit disorder. All do not have all of these traits any more than all have all the characteristics of ADD.

Desirable traits help protect the child against the ravages of the attention deficit disorder. Resiliency is one of their most profound defenses. Children with ADD may be daunted by negative feedback and momentary failures, but they keep coming back for more and frequently persist until objections or obstacles are overcome. Likewise, they usually do not hold grudges, but, rather, can be instantly forgiving. Most children with ADD are quite sensitive, as are adults with the condition. They are also often very intuitive and inquisitive. Their inquisitiveness may lead to destruction, but the intent is usually not malevolent. Rather, it is to see how things work. I remember, in days past, pediatricians used to collect objects that children had swallowed—everything from jacks to little toy cars to small tubes of glue. I collect records of things that children have taken apart.

A mother called me recently and asked me if I had a humidifier on the list. I had three: a Whirlpool and two GE's.

Many of these children, especially those with overactivity, have boundless energy and are indefatigable. Such energy can be a major asset if directed. ADD children are enthusiastic; they make great cheerleaders. Their attention to detail equips some well for being good draftsmen. Many have marvelous imaginations and may become good authors as long as a word processor is available. Many with ADD exhibit much emotional warmth and are not shy. They may be fun-loving with a good sense of humor and are often the life of the party. Many with ADD are acutely aware of their surroundings and have a remarkable memory for remote events. Those who have not developed too many oppositional behaviors are quite likeable. Good conversational ability is frequently found; and great salesmen and entrepreneurs abound among this group. If they learn to organize, many acquire wealth as well.

ADD children, adolescents and adults are usually more willing to take risks. Unlike the person with depression, they usually do not gunnysack their complaints or fortify their misery with events from the past. This is fortunate, for, over their lifetimes, many have experienced significant and, frequently, very negative consequences for their behaviors.

DESIRABLE TRAITS

- Resilient
- Accepting and forgiving
- Sensitive to the needs of others
- Inquisitive
- Intuitive
- Imaginative
- Boundless energy
- Good imagination
- Aware of detail
- Warm and fun-loving
- Good talkers
- Risk-takers

PART II

Diagnosing and Treating Attention Deficit Disorder

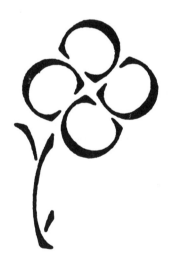

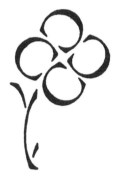

Diagnosis

We can diagnose attention deficit disorder if we understand attention deficit disorder, for to understand it is to diagnose it. There is no test for attention deficit disorder. Rather, it is a cluster of characteristics observed by parents and teachers. I remind you that Damon Runyon cautioned us to "Never ignore a tip from the jockey." In this case, the jockey is usually the mother or teacher. It has been shown repeatedly that if a mother or teacher brings you her concern, there is almost always a significant problem or misunderstanding. The fact that they have summoned up the courage to bring the concern to you should cause you to take them seriously.

Diagnosis is based on observation of the criteria listed as ADD characteristics in the DSM-III-R. It is important to remember that this is a pervasive disorder present over time and it may not be manifest unless the child is in his usual surroundings, certainly not the pediatrician or psychologist's office. It is often only manifest if the child is in the presence of structure and demands.

It is likely that before long there will be evidence to indicate that ADD can be differentiated from the mimics (LD, anxiety, depression) by neuropsychological testing of frontal lobe function. For test results to be reliable, the conditions of testing must include provisions for distraction. If the modifiers are present, test results will be skewed toward normalcy.

Remember the modifiers:

+ Novelty

+ Quiet environment

+ One-on-one interaction

+ Interesting

+ Repetitive feedback

+ Intimidation

+ Illness

The modifiers explain much of the mysterious fluctuation in performance characteristic of ADD. They may even make the disability disappear at times.

You must have the school records to assist you in making the diagnosis. You should have a record of at least two independent observations, preferably by parents and one or more teachers, who may, in their reports, record an entirely different story. That in itself is important. School is a structured environment with a great many demands that might not be made at home. Maybe the parents are relaxed and easy-going, and the child's hyperactive, boisterous behavior is of little concern to them. Maybe the teacher is too demanding, she has had little teaching experience, or she is intolerant of behaviors typical of those with ADD.

Behavior rating scales, though not absolutely necessary for the diagnosis, may be quite useful. I particularly like the *Copeland Symptom Checklist for ADD* and the *Achenbach Child Behavior Checklist (CBCL)*. The latter is a little more difficult to complete than the *Conners Rating Scales*, for it has 138 items. However, the CBCL includes a valuable section on social competence. This rating scale is not an attention deficit disorder diagnostic tool, but, rather, is used to assess a broad array of behaviors which may reveal or substantiate the presence of conditions which co-occur with the ADD or mimic it. A scale such as the Achenbach should be used if there is a family history of substance abuse, mental illness, sociopathic behavior, or physical or sexual abuse. It also should be used if the child exhibits significant oppositional behaviors, severe aggression or hallucinations.

George DuPaul, Ph.D., recently developed an ADHD rating scale using the characteristics in the DSM-III-R. This scale appears to be useful in ascertaining whether or not a child truly has skill-deficit behaviors characteristic of ADD. Numbers are assigned to the behaviors as *present a little, pretty much,* or *very much.* This scale I find to be of particular benefit in demonstrating the effectiveness of medication.[15]

The physical examination in youngsters with primary attention deficit disorder is usually unremarkable. I say *primary* to separate this condition from *acquired ADD* secondary to true brain damage, which may produce significant neurologic impairment.

Children with attention deficit disorder often exhibit some of the so-called neurologic soft signs which are of no great significance by themselves, but may fortify your contention that the child has attention deficit disorder. Some children without any abnormalities will exhibit these signs. These signs include difficulty in rapid alternating movements, overflow to the opposite extremity on sequential finger tapping, and hand drifting with arms outstretched. These signs represent persistence of immature movement patterns.

An EEG or MRI should only be done if history and physical examination suggest a seizure disorder or encephalopathy. A urine lead level should be obtained if there is question regarding the possibility of lead poisoning, or you are in an area where elevated lead levels are not uncommon.

The child under 12 and over 4 should have a complete visual-perceptual, visual-motor evaluation. Difficulty coloring within the lines often represents the ADD child's first academic failure.   Later, writing is described as *sloppy* or *messy*.   The presence of visual-motor perceptual deficits places the child at risk for problems in academic achievement.   There are two reasons for doing this evaluation.   One is to pick up a deficit co-morbidity that needs attention, and the other is to detect an at-risk indicator for learning disabilities.

It is a good idea to have a handle on the child's fine- and gross-motor ability, particularly in relation to handwriting, and to ascertain the potential for athletic prowess.   We're beginning to realize that quite a few children with attention deficit disorder exhibit deficiencies in motor planning, referred to as *dyspraxia*. Children with this difficulty often exhibit reluctance to enter a strange room and appear to be fearful.   They are trying to figure out how to motor plan their trip across unfamiliar territory.   Fine-motor dyspraxia may account for the clumsiness of their handwriting.

All children with attention deficit disorder should have a test of visual acuity and hearing competence, as well as an assessment of their abilities.   It is important that those working with the child be aware of the child's pattern of cognitive strengths and weaknesses.   The awareness of the impact of ADD on ability testing is also crucial since this disorder may markedly lower estimated intelligence[16].   Knowledge of a child's abilities is essential, not only to measure the discrepancy between measured intellectual ability and academic performance, which is a clue to learning disabilities, but also to help parents and teachers understand the degree to which a child's competencies can protect him against the difficulties of ADD.

In addition to the child's own unique talents and abilities, the protectors against the ravages of ADD include sincere, caring parent involvement; an appropriate, modified academic program; and peer- group acceptance.   Always look to the peer group, for it is the indicator as to how the child may function socially in adult life. The protection afforded by higher intelligence may not be as effective as the youngster moves into the more difficult work of high school.   This is the reason some have suggested *late-onset ADD*.   These children probably always had a discrepancy between ability and performance, but, being bright, they did not fail until high school or even college.   Some do not experience acute interference until graduate or professional school.

There are two children, one with an I.Q. of 90 and the other with an I.Q. of 120. Both have attention deficit disorder, and both have an ability to selectively attend to task for a period of ten minutes. Both are presented a problem. The child with the higher intelligence can solve the problem in eight minutes, within his span of attending ability, while the child with the lower I.Q. cannot get the answer to the problem within the time he's able to sustain his attention. If he could have paid attention for twelve minutes, he might well have come up with the right answer.

I recommend that children with diagnosed attention deficit disorder have a thorough learning disability evaluation. The child may not qualify for learning disability assistance, but all teachers who come in contact with the child should be thoroughly familiar with the child's learning strengths and weaknesses. Recognition of assets, difficulties and learning differences is important in the education and care of children with this condition. Testing of children with ADD reveals tremendous variability in performance. Achievement test profiles usually resemble the Himalayas. Achievement test scores, especially group measures, usually decline every year as long as the ADD remains untreated.

Having both an attention deficit disorder and a learning disability is a double whammy and makes the goal of providing appropriate education more difficult. Don't assume the ADD child has LD until after treatment for the ADD has been instituted. Sometimes academic difficulties due to ADD can look very much like learning disabilities.

If I am certain the child has ADD, I request that the child's school provide a learning disability evaluation, including intelligence testing. I rely upon a developmentally-trained occupational therapist for a perceptual-motor and motor-planning evaluation and a skilled audiologist and optometrist to test hearing and vision, respectively.

In arriving at an appropriate diagnosis, the presence of emotional or psychiatric disorders must be determined. If present, they must be treated as a co-morbidity. Some psychiatrists feel that the presence of anxiety or true depression are contraindications to the use of medications traditionally employed in the treatment of attention deficit disorder (Ritalin, Dexedrine and Cylert—the psychostimulants). Others do not agree.

DIAGNOSIS

- Diagnosis is based on the history and observations of parents and teachers. Physicians and mental health professionals interpret the data and exclude other disorders that can affect attention.

- Behavior rating scales are useful, particularly if the history suggests the child to be at risk for a mimic or co-morbidity. They are also helpful in determining areas of greatest difficulty, and for monitoring medication effects.

- Physical and laboratory examinations are of little help except when specifically indicated.

- Visual-motor perceptual testing should be done.

- Gross- and fine-motor ability should be evaluated.

- Check for developmental dyspraxia.

- Vision and hearing should be examined.

- The child should be given an I.Q. test.

- LD evaluation should be carried out.

- Emotional or psychiatric disorders must be excluded.

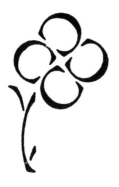

Multimodal Treatment

For attention deficit disorder, there is no cure. It is a complex problem which cannot be fixed by eliminating sugar or food coloring or by any other simple solution. Someone once said, "For every truly complex problem there is always a simple solution which is direct, succinct, brief, and wrong." This is a developmental disability for which there is no cure, but there is a considerable amount of help.

Effective treatment cannot be provided by a single modality, whether medication, educational intervention or behavior management. All are necessary. The treatment of the condition is multimodal. It is imperative that we treat by inventory and not by diagnosis. You don't say, "Okay, he has attention deficit disorder, we'll put this plan into action." You look at all the characteristics of the disorder, taking all assets and liabilities into account. Some children are more impulsive, while others are more distractible. Some have a severe deficit in attending ability, but are not particularly overactive. Some are underactive and even lethargic.

All characteristics fit somewhere on the bell-shaped curve. Your job is to determine where and how helpful or detrimental the degree of its presence will be to the child's success. No two youngsters with attention deficit disorder are alike. Take an inventory of the child's strengths and weaknesses and treat accordingly. The goal of your care and intervention with this child is to improve the goodness of fit between her environment and the characteristics of her disorder so that she experiences the best possible quality of life.

◆ ◆ ◆ ◆ ◆ ◆

TREATMENT

◆ Education.

◆ Medication.

◆ Application of . . .

  • academic modifications.
  • behavior management.

◆ Treat by inventory, not by diagnosis.

◆ All characteristics fall somewhere on the bell-shaped curve. Their positions determine the remedial efforts needed.

◆ The goal of treatment is to improve the goodness of fit so that there is a good quality of life.

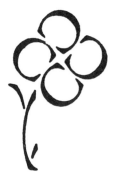

Education of Parents,
Teachers and Children

To understand attention deficit disorder is to diagnose it. To understand the condition is to treat it.

Treating attention deficit disorder effectively requires, first, a thorough understanding of the biologic nature of the condition; its characteristics and ramifications; and its effects on family life, school performance and self-image. This can only be accomplished by a willingness on the part of parents and teachers to become informed, and on the part of the physician to educate. You should provide families with current, factual, understandable, instructional literature, and you must assess their knowledge of it. (See Appendices B and C for suggestions regarding instructional material.)

Before there is any plan of treatment employed, all involved must be educated. We're talking about parent education, not parenting classes. Most of these parents can parent a child without attention deficit disorder quite adequately and have done so. Teachers need education, too, for most teachers have not learned a significant amount about attention deficit disorder in their education courses. Don't ever blame the teacher for a lack of knowledge. It is our obligation to help teachers understand. It is important that we all become advocates for children, not adversaries of the school system. Good teachers welcome information, for it is their heartfelt desire to see to it that the child's academic performance is commensurate with the child's learning abilities.

The child must also be educated regarding ADD, even though he may wonder, "What's all this fuss about?" To maintain a good self-image, he needs to recognize his liabilities, as well as his assets. He must recognize what the disability means to him and must know there are ways he can be helped. We can often assist in the maintenance of self-esteem by pointing out to the child that, considering the nature of his disability, his performance is commendable. (See Appendix B for literature that is helpful in educating the child about ADD.)

♦ ♦ ♦ ♦ ♦ ♦

EDUCATE

♦ Parents

♦ Teachers

♦ The child with ADD

Medication

The majority of children with attention deficit disorder will benefit significantly from the employment of replacement therapy, *i.e.,* replacing a deficient chemical in order to improve performance. By so doing, we bring the child's attending ability closer to that of children without ADD and assist the child in improving other incompetent ADD behaviors.

Over one million children with ADD in the United States are being treated with psychostimulants. Over one hundred and fifty carefully controlled studies speak to the effectiveness of these agents. I will primarily write about Ritalin, for Ritalin (generic: *methylphenidate hydrochloride*) makes up about 85% of the prescriptions for attention deficit disorder. What I say about Ritalin will generally apply to the other psychostimulants, dextroamphetamine sulfate (*Dexedrine*), and magnesium pemoline (*Cylert*). I will point out the differences between Ritalin and the other medications when I briefly discuss them later in this section.

Attempts to synthesize ephedrine in the laboratory resulted in the discovery of amphetamine (Benzedrine), the right-hand form of which is dextroamphetamine (Dexedrine). While experimenting with amphetamine, a scientist attached a piperidine ring and a new compound called *methylphenidate hydrochloride* was produced. This is why the initials *MPH* are sometimes used for generic Ritalin. The de-esterification of MPH results in an inactive metabolite, *ritalinic acid*, hence the name *Ritalin*.

Ritalin and the other stimulant medications presumably improve attending by enhancing the efficacy of dopamine, which improves the regulation of attention, impulsivity, and extraneous movement. When prescribing Ritalin, I initially recommend a 2.5 mg. dose in the morning and 2.5 mg. dose at noon in the child under 60 pounds, and 5 mg. in the morning, 5 mg. at noon in the child over 60 pounds. Starting with low doses often negates the appearance of bothersome side effects. I prefer to first prescribe, taking the medication early morning and approximately four hours later, for I am initially interested in enhancing performance at school and wish to avoid the remote possibility of sleeping difficulties from Ritalin given later in the day. Continuing the medication on weekends improves efficient monitoring and dose adjustment.

The effect of Ritalin therapy is not dependent upon a mg./kg. dose. Body weight has little influence on the amount of medication necessary to obtain a clinical response. The medication has a high affinity for certain areas of the brain and is taken up almost immediately. This is why outcome studies employing various doses, such as .3 mg./kg. versus .8 mg/kg. are of little value. You adjust the dose according to clinical response observed by parents and teachers. The child himself may not be aware of a change. In some children, a 5 mg. dose will be as effective as a 20 mg. dose in another child the same size. Neither is the dose employed dependent upon the severity of the ADD. Five milligrams two to three times a day may adequately treat both mild and severe ADD.

The effect of Ritalin usually appears within 15 to 20 minutes, peaks at approximately 2 hours and lasts for a period of 3 to 5 hours, usually about 4. There is no cumulative effect. This is an important recognition. You are basically providing medical therapy for four-hour periods of time, although, in some children, the effect will last as long as six hours, and in some no more than two hours. The lack of a cumulative effect contributes to the safety of the medication and is the characteristic which renders weaning the child off the medication unnecessary.

Often it is beneficial to give a dose at 4 p.m., especially as homework demands increase, or the child becomes involved in demanding after-school activities such as team sports or music lessons. It is not unusual for some children to experience a hyperactive rebound about 4 p.m. as the effect of the medication wears off. Should this be the case, first reduce the noon dose. If that is not effective, consider giving a 4 p.m. dose. The afternoon dose may be less than the morning or noon dose.

An important effect of the medication is to make the child more receptive to education and behavior management. We must recognize, however, that Ritalin is not a behavior pill. While Ritalin does help impulsive behavior, it does not eliminate oppositional, defiant behaviors. The child must be held accountable for these actions and managed accordingly.

The target response is attending, not defiant behavior. Handwriting often improves, but it may not. Yes, the child might not be so physically active, and yes, he might not be quite so impulsive. All are beneficial effects, but the target response is the child's ability to attend. It is important to remember this, for I have seen youngsters with oppositional defiant behaviors with very significant attending problems, placed on Ritalin and teachers and others said that it was of no benefit. The oppositional defiant behavior continued, even though the attending ability was better. This benefit may be overlooked if the child continues to be difficult.

Gradually, every two to four weeks, I increase the dose of Ritalin until effect is apparent. It is generally not necessary to exceed 20 mg. three to four times a day. If the medication is beneficial, you will know it. So will the piano teacher and the parish priest. There will be change when you use this medication if the diagnosis is correct. If there is no change, the physician should realize that not enough medication is being prescribed. Without this realization it is common never to reach a therapeutic level and to consider the medication ineffective. When some clinical effect is evident, but there is not a fairly dramatic response, I will increase the dose, hoping for a more favorable outcome. If symptoms of overdose appear, I reduce the dose until they disappear. If there is an adverse response, I will try another psychostimulant until I have utilized all three.

Do not employ *drug holidays.* I deplore the term. I have never used it. It doesn't quite make sense to bring to the child the connotation that, "Whoopie doo, you're on a holiday, you don't have to take that medicine." It is this drug-holiday sort of attitude that I am sure sends an inappropriate message to parents and teachers. I have heard of teachers giving a party in their classrooms to celebrate with holiday spirit the fact that Jason or Charles no longer has to take his "behavior pill."

We must insist on compliance. If I detect, despite considerable effort, noncompliance on the part of parents, school personnel, or the older patient himself, I will discontinue the medication. We should attempt to avoid the yo-yo effect, for consistency is so important in dealing with a child with attention deficit disorder. School personnel must give the medication and not leave compliance up to the child. The school, not the child, should be responsible for seeing to it that the medication is taken. The school is legally obligated under Section 504 of P.L. 93-112 (the Rehabilitation Act) to administer medication appropriately and document their having done so.[17]

The child should have the medication if he benefits from the medication. He should have it if the medication assists in improving the fit between the child's disability and the nature of his environment. This is true on weekends as well as during the week. It is true in summer as well as during the school year. In ascertaining this goodness of fit, constantly look at the demands placed upon the child. At times, if the demands are less, such as they might be during the summer, the child may be able to operate effectively without medication, providing there is no significant deterioration in psychosocial adjustment as measured by peer-group acceptance and family harmony. In considering the goodness of fit, let's not forget interpersonal relationships and social competence. If the medication improves the child's acceptance by others, the medication is indicated. Rejection is a very unhealthy negative consequence. Acceptance by the peer group is essential in maintaining one's good feelings about oneself. Peer-group acceptance is well documented as one of the best ways of protecting the child against an undesirable outcome.

It is best not to allow the child to start school in the fall without medication. A new school year, usually with a new teacher and different demands, is particularly difficult for a child with ADD. Transitions always present problems. If the child has not been on medication over the summer, I usually start the medicine two weeks before the beginning of school.

♦ *Ritalin SR*

There is a sustained release form of Ritalin, *Ritalin SR-20*, which has gotten perhaps more bad press than fully deserved. A long-acting medication is often advantageous to attempt to avoid the noon-time trip to the school office as the child gets older. In the majority of cases, there will be a clinically effective blood level for six to eight hours. It is a slow-release medication; therefore, it may be too slow in the mornings. Should this be the case, I prescribe from 5 to 10 mg. of regular Ritalin along with the early morning SR dose. If the child is getting only six hours of benefit from the SR, a second dose in the afternoon can be helpful. If coverage is needed beginning about 1:00 to 2:00 p.m., I would advise another SR dose. If coverage is not required until approximately 3:00 to 4:00 p.m., regular Ritalin avoids the possibility of sleep interference. Different regimens are tried until optimum benefit has been achieved.

Ritalin SR is more expensive, the opportunity to treat discrete four-hour episodes of life and valuable flexibility are lost, and it is available only in one dosage form, a white 20 mg. tablet. Regular Ritalin comes in scored 5 mg. yellow, 10 mg. light blue and 20 mg. larger yellow tablets. Some children may have a hyperkinetic, hypersensitivity reaction to the number 10 yellow dye in 5 and 20 mg. tablets. A common mistake in prescribing Ritalin SR is giving inadequate doses. While SR-20 is supposed to equal 10 mg. of regular Ritalin taken twice daily, in practice it is the equivalent of approximately 7½ mg. twice a day. Approximately 20% more SR than the total daily dose of regular Ritalin must be given for comparable results. For example, if a child is responding to 15 mg. in the morning and at noon, then he will, in all probability, require two 20 mg. SR tablets in the morning.

The advisability of using generic Ritalin (methylphenidate) is often raised as an issue. I use it, for it is cheaper and is effective in the vast majority of cases when one understands the potential problems with its use. To comply with the law, the desired action and correct chemical formulation must be present in the generic compound of any drug. However, approximately 25% tolerance on either side of the dose level, called "*The Rule of 75*," is allowed in the amount of effective agent in generic compounds. Often the apparent non-response to a generic is because the child is getting 25% less of the active ingredient. A dose adjustment may solve the problem. Occasionally, a batch of generic methylphenidate will not be effective at a dose that previously worked. If that occurs, try a different generic or change to the Ciba Geigy brand Ritalin.

♦ *Dexedrine*

Some physicians prefer Dexedrine as their drug of choice. I do not. I am with the majority who favor Ritalin. Dexedrine, however, may be effective when Ritalin is not. Ritalin, likewise, may be effective when Dexedrine is not. Regular Dexedrine comes in a 5 mg. orange triangular-shaped tablet and usually will be effective for a period of 3-4 hours.

Dexedrine is becoming my drug of choice in attention deficit disorder without hyperactivity. This condition is called *Undifferentiated Attention Deficit Disorder*. This classification may disappear from the next DSM, just as attention deficit disorder with hypoactivity disappeared. Or it may be classified as *Cognitive Attention Deficit Disorder* and included in the Learning Disabilities category of disorders. DSM-IV is currently being written with a planned publishing date of 1994.

It is possible that many children with attention deficit disorder without hyperactivity have significant cerebral processing dysfunction. These are the children who are sometimes referred to as *space cadets*. They don't pay attention because they are having difficulty processing auditory and/or visual information, especially auditory input. Some of these youngsters appear to demonstrate better attending ability and improvement in their cognitive processing abilities when given Dexedrine. There may possibly be a preference in this instance over Ritalin.

There is a long-acting form of Dexedrine, *Dexedrine Spansule*, which is reported to be effective for 6 to 8 hours, depending on individual metabolism. It is available in 5 mg., 10 mg., and 15 mg. capsules. Dexedrine Spansule is worthy of consideration when either the effects of Ritalin or regular Dexedrine are lasting no more than two to three hours and several doses must be given during the day. In this situation the spansule form of Dexedrine may have effects that last 4 to 6 hours and two doses a day are usually sufficient. Some consider Dexedrine in spansule form a better long-acting medication than Ritalin SR.

Dexedrine and Ritalin are not milligram-for-milligram equivalent. Often a smaller dose of Dexedrine, usually two-thirds to one-half, can be given to obtain the same results. Dexedrine Spansule is formulated differently from Ritalin SR with some of the medication in the capsule being in the regular fast-acting form. This formulation has the advantage of providing more rapid morning coverage. Some children are very aware of the short-acting medications' peak-and-valley effect. These children often prefer the smoother effect of a long-acting medication. The long-acting medications also may have a much diminished rebound effect.

I usually do not use Dexedrine as my first choice, for it is considered a *street drug*. Potential for abuse appears greater, not by the child with the attention deficit disorder, but by other members of the family, especially adolescents. In addition, I find that there is more appetite-suppressant effect from Dexedrine than from Ritalin and, in general, more undesirable minor side effects, although that has not been the experience of some others. It is a helpful second-choice medication in my practice and does not have any more significant side effects than Ritalin.

◆ *Cylert*

Another medication used for attention deficit disorder is magnesium pemoline or Cylert. I use it on occasion when, for one reason or another, Dexedrine and Ritalin are not options. Occasionally you will find that Cylert is effective when the other two are not. In some children, it is extremely effective. Its advantages include its long-acting effect so that, usually, it can be given in a single morning dose. It is not a Class II drug, so you can give a refillable prescription or phone it in to the pharmacy. Prescriptions for Ritalin and Dexedrine must follow stringent state guidelines which differ somewhat from state to state. Generally, prescriptions must be in writing, filled within 2-7 days of the date on the prescription, and only a limited supply can be prescribed at one time.

The most significant disadvantage of Cylert is that it does not have a readily discernable time of onset and termination of effect. It may take two to three weeks after initiation of therapy before the optimum clinical effect of the medication is apparent, although some improvement may be noted within a few days. A gradually diminishing effect may last for days to weeks after it is discontinued. Because its effectiveness depends on maintaining a continuous therapeutic blood level, it cannot be discontinued on weekends or holidays. Another disadvantage for children are the periodic blood tests which are advised.

It is estimated that Cylert will work well in approximately 30% of children with ADD. The usual minimum effective dose is 56.75 mg., and 75 mg. is average. It comes in strange amounts per tablet of 18.75 mg. and 37.5 mg. Fortunately, 75 mg., the dose most often required, comes in a pill which contains that amount. There is also a chewable 37.5 mg. tablet.

Cylert has some unusual side effects not seen with Ritalin and Dexedrine. The incidence of rash is higher and lip-biting and finger-picking may be side effects. Some youngsters get marked excoriation around their mouths from scraping their lips with their teeth. I have had a few patients on Cylert who have experienced a non-cardiac-related vibratory sensation in their chest. In addition, Cylert can occasionally cause liver impairment. It is recommended that liver function tests be obtained every three to six months. Cylert, unlike Ritalin and Dexedrine, may exhibit tachyphylaxis and become less effective as time goes on.

♦ *Monitoring Medication*

After diagnosis, and with the onset of medical intervention, I request that both parents and child attend a six-week video-facilitated group therapeutic/educational program. At each group session, I monitor and adjust the medication of each child, educate parents and child in various aspects of ADD and address the emotional issues and impact the disorder has had, and will have on each member of the family. This program has proved extremely effective in ensuring adequate monitoring and follow-through of medication, and in providing for the therapeutic and educational needs of both the parents and child. A great benefit for the physician is the bonding which occurs with the family, the greatly reduced number of phone calls received, and the time required to answer parents' questions. If the family cannot, due to distance or other reasons, attend the weekly sessions, I see the child and at least one parent every two to four weeks.

I request that the parent make contact with the teacher for a report on school progress and the effectiveness of medication prior to each visit. I find that if I require parents to do this, the all-important communication link between school and home is improved. I use these visits to increase the family's knowledge about ADD and to question both parents and child regarding what they have learned about the condition. It is also an opportunity to provide positive reinforcement to parents and child. Medication is adjusted according to clinical response and the presence or absence of side effects. To this end, I often request that behavioral, attending, and side-effect checklists be completed by parents and teachers.

Once an appropriate dose and regimen are achieved for a particular child, I schedule visits every three months. Such monitoring is critical. During these visits I always check height and weight and review the growth chart with the child and parents. The child's blood pressure is recorded and the quality of motor movement is determined by requiring a finger-to-nose test, sequential finger tapping, and an observation of rapid alternating movements by pronation and supination of the outstretched arms. Behavioral, attending, and side-effects checklists completed by both parents and teachers are reviewed.

I'm often asked, "How long will my child have to take medication?" My response is that he doesn't have to take it at all. He will not become severely ill or endanger his physical well being if he does not take the medication. On the other hand, the medication will, in all likelihood, significantly improve the quality of his life and, as long as it does, it is prudent to take it. The choice is the family's.

The average duration of medication in my practice is four to five years, during which time the medication assists the child in developing his own skills so that he can cope effectively with his condition. After one to two years, I usually give the child a trial off medication during the school year, always waiting at least a week for psychological adjustment before making the decision to resume the medication or not. The child must never look upon continuation of medication as a defeat. Again a word of caution—please do not try the child off of medication at the beginning of a new school year. Wait until she has successfully adjusted and then do so. Late winter or early spring are good times. Don't do it over Christmas vacation, for there is too much distracting excitement. Holidays off medication can be exceedingly difficult for child and family and serve no real purpose.

These medications, properly used, are remarkable in their ability to improve the ADD child's life with a minimum of risk. However, they cannot do it all. They cannot correct oppositional and other negative or inappropriate behaviors which can only effectively be changed with appropriate behavioral interventions. Stimulant medication for the child with attention deficit disorder can reasonably be expected to . . .

Increase:
- tolerance
- sustained attention
- solitary play

Decrease:
- impulsivity
- task-irrelevant physical activity
- boredom

They usually improve handwriting, academic performance, peer relations, extracurricular activities and family interactions as well.

◆ *Contraindications*

Contraindications to the use of these medications include glaucoma and high blood pressure. Some feel that affective and mood disorders are contraindications. Others do not agree, but speak to the judicious use of stimulant medications in these conditions. Some may use Ritalin or Dexedrine for the attention deficit disorder combined with another medication for anxiety or depression. This practice is becoming more common, especially the use of Tofranil (imipramine), usually 25-50 mg., at bedtime to decrease moodiness and irritability, while the stimulant medication is used during the day for attention and focused behavior. Bipolar disorders can be treated with Ritalin and Lithium combined, but this intervention is tricky and best left to psychiatrists. If the child's family history includes Bipolar or Manic-Depressive Disorder, one should be alert to the possible presence of it in the child. These issues are addressed in some detail in *Medications for Attention Disorders (ADHD/ADD) and Related Medical Problems: A Comprehensive Handbook* listed in Appendix C.

The stimulant drugs, Ritalin, Dexedrine and Cylert, are not addictive when used in the treatment of ADD, nor is there evidence to suggest that their use leads to addiction in later life. Many have suggested that, because of the better self-image that results from the proper use of these medications, subsequent drug addiction is less common in those with ADD who are medically and behaviorally treated than in those who go untreated.

It is always important in your work with the child with ADD to emphasize that the child is receiving replacement therapy and that *he*, not the medication, is in control. Good behavior must never be attributed to the medication. Subsequent to bad behavior, no one should say, "You must have forgotten to take your pill," or "Did you take your medicine?" Both parents and teachers must be forewarned against making this ever-so-common, understandable but potentially quite detrimental mistake.

These medications, properly used, do not alter the child's basic personality. They will not preclude boisterous, active behavior when such behavior is appropriate. There is no diminution of freedom of expression, curiosity, imagination or creativity when children with ADD take these medications. They may, however, be less funny with their classmates, especially if they have found an acceptable role with their peers as the "class clown."

◆ *Side Effects*

There are few serious side effects. The psychostimulants are remarkably safe. They have been used for many, many years, so I am comfortable making that statement. Dexedrine was used in the 30's and the use of Ritalin began shortly thereafter. Dexedrine was first used as an appetite suppressant and a mood elevator. Ritalin was primarily used to treat chronic fatigue syndrome.

A few years ago I was asked to appear on a television program to give my impressions of a TV appearance of a lawyer who made the statement, "Ritalin must be banned." This lawyer represented the Citizens Commission on Human Rights. It sounds as if objecting to a *commission on human rights* is like speaking in opposition to motherhood or the flag. The Citizens Commission on Human Rights is sponsored by the Church of Scientology, which, in this country, represents the last bastion of Ritalin objectors. One of the statements I made on that program was, "Serious side effects from Ritalin are less common than serious side effects from Penicillin." This is a true statement.

I have yet to see a serious side effect from Ritalin over the twenty years I have used it. Serious side effects include dystonic movement disorders and *tardive dyskinesia*, a catatonic-like rigidity of movement which may be permanent. There are only a few cases in the world's literature, and it is my understanding that these reports concerned adults who had been on the medication for many years. Occasionally in an adult, and rarely in an adolescent, this medication can precipitate an acute psychotic episode. This reaction, though rare, has caused some to shun the use of stimulant medications in adults. Those more knowledgeable use them as long as they differentiate the signs and symptoms of attention deficit disorder from serious psychotic disturbances such as schizophrenia and bipolar disorders. It appears that most, if not all, who have had acute psychotic episodes as a consequence of Ritalin and similar medications have been found to have significant psychiatric disorders which were exacerbated by the use of this medication.

There are relatively common minor side effects. Decreased appetite is seen in approximately 60% of cases but, for most, is not severe and does not last more than a week or two. When there is severe depression of appetite early on, it serves as a clue that you will probably not be able to use the medication because of persistent anorexia. Any deleterious effect on growth appears related more to inadequate nutrition as a consequence of appetite suppression than to suppression of growth hormones. This area, however, continues to be investigated. These medications, in dosages typically prescribed, seem to have no direct effect on growth in most children.

Insomnia and sleep disturbance can occur. Some children may experience special difficulty falling asleep if bedtime coincides with the time the effect of the medication is wearing off. It is not uncommon to find that late afternoon or early evening Ritalin, in smaller doses, may have a beneficial effect on sleep. Sleep machines, such as an inexpensive one available from Sears, are helpful to many children, especially those with hearing sensitivity and those quite auditorially distracted, for episodic noises often keep them awake. Fans and vaporizers can serve the same purpose by providing a consistent low level of noise.

Mild abdominal periumbilical discomfort is common. If this should occur, especially if combined with appetite suppression, it is best to give the Ritalin with meals. Digestive juices do not interfere with absorption, as suggested in the early 80's. Mild headaches are common initially, usually responding adequately to simple medications such as ibuprofen or acetaminophen. Whiny, irritable behavior concerns me. I do not like to see it. This is the most common, really bothersome, side effect that I encounter. If these symptoms persist and do not respond immediately to dose reduction, I discontinue the medication. If there is any personality change, the medication should be decreased or discontinued. Some children appear sad on the medication. I don't like to see this either but usually this is a transient dysphoria. If it persists, I will discontinue the medication. Dizziness, dry mouth, constipation, rashes and nausea are rare. High blood pressure is pretty unusual though not quite so rare. I have seen hair loss on three occasions, the hair returning with discontinuation of the medication. Nightmares may be a complication of medication for ADD, while night terrors are characteristic of the condition.

When receiving too much medication, the child may become lethargic. However, he is more likely to become sullen, withdrawn, irritable and/or twitchy. I have never witnessed the *zombie-like* state described by Ritalin objectors. If one did, one would, of course, immediately change one's prescriptive advice. It is hard to imagine that any physician would allow a child to continue in such a state without altering the medication. This response is probably not a medication side effect, but rather occurs as a consequence of too much medication. Overdosing is often secondary to a physician attempting erroneously to control defiant oppositional behavior with a psychostimulant, or increasing the dosage when the medication is not effective as a result of the wrong diagnosis.

Some children on medication will develop facial tics and grimacing. This may or may not be an early sign of Tourette Syndrome (TS). Often children with TS will present with attention deficit disorder and/or learning disabilities long before other manifestations of the condition. At one time it was believed by many that the use of Ritalin, Dexedrine or Cylert was contraindicated if tics should appear. Most who are familiar with these conditions will often continue to advise the use of these effective medications under close supervision, and may use them in conjunction with other medications, if there is marked improvement in the attentional deficits on the medication. These practitioners, including myself, will not deny a youngster with some tics and facial grimacing the beneficial effects of these medications. In some instances, the risk is well worth it. It is estimated that the use of psychostimulants will increase tics in half of Tourette Syndrome patients.[18]   Parents should be told that continued use of the medications might worsen tics and may even hasten the appearance of other Tourette's symptoms, such as uncontrolled explosive vocal utterances, though, at present, this is conjecture.

If tics should worsen to the point that they disrupt the child's life, then an alternate medication such as desipramine (*Norpramin*) may be tried in post-pubertal children/teens. Imipramine (*Tofranil*), however, may exacerbate tics. Desipramine is usually not as effective as the psychostimulants in altering the manifestations of ADD, but it may have some beneficial effect and is not reported to exaggerate tics. Clonidine (*Catapres*) has been used by some for those with tics, but I find it to be relatively ineffective in treating ADD unless utilized in conjunction with a smaller dose of stimulant medication. Dexedrine has been reported to be somewhat less likely to exacerbate tics than Ritalin, but others disagree.

Orange juice and other acid foods will interfere with the absorption of Dexedrine, while antihistamines will reduce the effectiveness of both Ritalin and Dexedrine.   Both of these medications may increase the blood levels of anticonvulsants. A seizure disorder is not a contraindication to the use of the psychostimulants, but medication should be monitored carefully when stimulants are part of the medical management of the child.

Stimulant medications are usually less effective in the very young. They generally are not employed in children under five years of age, although I occasionally do so, especially with very impulsive, hyperactive children and hyperactive children with language disorders. When used in younger children, it is more difficult to titrate clinical response. It is not uncommon to fail to observe any beneficial effects from these medications in young children.   You may even see increases in hyperactivity and impulsivity only to find the medications very beneficial when the child is older. Central nervous system maturation appears to be a factor. If a parent says to you that Dexedrine was tried when the child was three and it "made him worse," don't hesitate to give either Ritalin or Dexedrine a trial if the child has obvious attention deficit disorder and is now 7 or 8 years of age.

Few children with true ADD will fail to respond to Ritalin. The decision to change to another medication is usually dictated by the appearance of undesirable side effects rather than a lack of clinical response. At times, inappropriate medication is given to a child who has been misdiagnosed.

If you are certain the child has ADD and no significant mental or emotional illness, exhaust all possible avenues for prescribing psychostimulants. These agents are more likely to ameliorate incompetent ADD behaviors than any other medical or psychological intervention. Tricyclic antidepressants, by contrast, are more complicated to use, have more serious side effects and usually are not as effective.

◆ *Other Medications*

Other psychoactive agents which are designed to affect mood and behavior are sometimes used in children with attention deficit disorder. They include the tricyclic antidepressants (TCAs), imipramine (*Tofranil*), desipramine (*Norpramin*), and other antidepressants.

Mellaril, a neuroleptic drug, is a tranquilizer used especially in younger children with severe oppositional aggressive behaviors. Haloperidol (*Haldol*) and pimozide (*Orap*) are often used for Tourette Syndrome and may, at times, be utilized in TS in conjunction with the psychostimulants, reducing the tic manifestations worsened by Ritalin. Some children with TS will respond to clonidine (*Catapres*) with a reduction of tics and impaired attending. It is safer than either Haldol or Orap. Fluoxetine (*Prozac*) has not been effective in the treatment of ADD, although it has been used successfully with stimulant medications in older adolescents and adults to treat co-morbidities such as depression or obsessive-compulsive disorder (OCD). Some have reported a worsening of ADD symptoms on this medication. A possible exception to avoiding the use of Prozac in children concerns a specific type of attention difficulty seen at times in children with Tourette Syndrome. Most children with TS, who have difficulty attending, have a deficit characteristic of true ADD. Some, however, may have a deficit in attention that is related to obsessive compulsive disorder. This may be more common than originally perceived. They are so overfocused on details that they do not attend to the whole. Prozac has been reported to be of benefit for this group of children. Clomipramin (*Anafranil*), another TCA, is also used for OCD. It must be given with meals, for it often causes nausea.

The tricyclic antidepressants have gained some popularity in the treatment of ADD. These agents block the re-uptake of norepinephrine. They are the medications of choice if the stimulants are contraindicated because of side effects. They are also used by many as drugs of choice in the child with ADD who is anxious or depressed. However, currently many physicians in this situation use the psychostimulants to treat the ADD symptoms along with the tricyclics or other medications for anxiety or depression. For the child without ADD, who has some ADD-like symptoms caused by anxiety or depression, these medications can be quite effective. It has been suggested that imipramine may be more effective in anxiety, while desipramine is more effective in depression. Desipramine has not been approved for use in children under age 12.

Most pediatricians prefer imipramine, for they are more familiar with its use over many years. I begin with an evening dose of 10 mg. in the child under 50 pounds, and 25 mg. in the child over 50 pounds, increasing gradually. Generally an effective dose ranges from 2 to 3 mg/kg, but doses as high as 4-5 mg/kg have been used. In order to reduce peak effect, it is advisable to give a split evening-morning dosage when 3 mg/kg or more is prescribed.

The common side effects of the TCAs result from their anticholinergic effect—dry mouth leading to dental carries, blurred vision, constipation and urinary retention.

All avenues of dosage, medication form, and timing of psychostimulant medication should be explored before considering the use of the antidepressants which are not as safe and generally not as effective for the treatment of ADD. In my opinion, if you entertain the use of these agents for any reason other than the inability of the child to take the stimulants due to intolerable side effects, you should refer the child to a psychiatrist well versed in treating ADD. I encourage you to do so, for in this event it is quite probable that the child has a significant co-morbidity or that you have misdiagnosed the condition.

The risk of using these agents is greater than for the psychostimulants. This is especially true of desipramine in prepubescent children in whom three cardiac deaths have been reported. It is advised that an EKG rhythm strip be obtained as a baseline to rule out preexisting cardiac conduction defects, then again when the maintenance dose is reached whenever imipramine or desipramine is used. In addition, the potential for serious consequences as a result of overdose far exceeds that for the psychostimulants. Incidentally, bedwetting in the ADD child is not considered a good rationale for using imipramine, a tricyclic antidepressant, rather than a psychostimulant. The tricyclic antidepressants, in doses employed for ADD, are potentially more harmful and are less likely to be effective. A third dose of Ritalin has been found to have beneficial effects on bedwetting in some children.

Buspirone (*Buspar*) is an excellent antianxiety agent with fewer side effects than other such agents. It comes in 5 and 10 mg. tablets. The average dose in adults and older children is 20 to 30 mg. t.i.d.

Buproprion (*Wellbutrin*), because of its effects on the re-uptake of norepinephrine and dopamine, has been utilized by some who believed it to be effective for depression as well as ADD. It certainly is not as effective as the psychostimulants for ADD, and few will chance its use, for significant numbers of persons have experienced grand mal seizures while taking Wellbutrin. A flu-like illness, with nausea, vomiting and diarrhea, is a relatively common side effect and nocturia, edema, ataxia and stomatitis have been reported.

Nortriptyline (*Pamelor*) has been used by some to treat ADD. It is a good antidepressant, but apparently is not as effective as the other tricyclics in treating ADD. It has not been approved for use in children. The generally effective dose is 75-100 mg. per day either t.i.d. or as a single night-time dose. If over 100 mg/day is used, blood levels must be obtained. The therapeutic range is considered to be 50-150 ng/ml. Liver function studies are necessary, for a chemical hepatitis has been reported.

I would not prescribe any of the nonstimulant agents without serious study of the psychopharmacology involved—side effects and risks—being particularly aware of cardiac complications.

I have not had significant success in using clonidine (Catapres) in the treatment of ADD but do find that it is often effective when used in conjunction with Ritalin in reducing rage outbursts in those children who have what is referred to as *dyscontrol*. Ritalin is used to improve the ADD skill deficits while clonidine has the effect of improving the brain's inhibition of wild, out-of-control behavior. Also used in dyscontrol are propranolol, *Inderal*, which has fewer side effects but is less effective, and *Tegretol*. Tegretol, an anticonvulsant, is effective in some children with rage outbursts, especially those with mental retardation and/or organic brain pathology. Tegretol is not used to treat ADD *per se*, but may be quite effective in treating rage outbursts occurring with or without an EEG abnormality.

♦ *Clonidine*

Clonidine (Catapres) is an antihypertensive agent which has been found to have central nervous system effects related to inhibition. It currently is widely prescribed in programs designed to stop smoking. The primary side effects are lethargy, which is often quite profound, and hypotension. A 10% fall in systolic blood pressure is not uncommon on even small doses.

Clonidine comes in 0.1 mg., 0.2 mg. and 0.3 mg. tablets and a cutaneous long-acting patch, which is great for smokers who want to quit if their skin doesn't become sensitive to it. Children with ADD rarely keep the patch in place. Because lethargy is such a common side effect, medication should be started at night in a small dose. In initiating therapy, I usually choose one-fourth or one-half of a 0.1 mg. tablet at bedtime. After about a week, I increase to one-half to one 0.1 mg. tablet at night and a week later, if all is well, add a morning dose of .05 mg. (one-half tablet). If the child becomes lethargic, I increase by only one-fourth tablet. Once I'm able to attain a dose morning and night, I will add a mid-day dose, for clonidine t.i.d. medication appears to be a more effective regimen than twice daily. The secret of appropriate application of clonidine therapy is to use small amounts often. It may take as long as one to two months of gradual increase in dose to arrive at a clinically effective level without undue lethargy. In children with severe episodic out-of-control behavior, the wait is often worth it. No behavior- management technique in the world will be effective in these cases.

It is important to point out that rebound hypertension has been reported following sudden withdrawal of this medication. Clonidine should be withdrawn gradually to avoid a potentially dangerous increase in blood pressure, and withdrawal symptoms of headache, nausea and agitation.

Medication should be a concomitant contribution to multimodal treatment and not a last resort if all else fails. If theory is correct, and there is much evidence to suggest that it is, medication will help to normalize brain chemistry.

♦ ♦ ♦ ♦ ♦ ♦

MEDICATION

♦ Ritalin makes up 85% of the prescriptions for ADD.

♦ Approximately one million children with ADD are being treated with psychostimulants and the number is increasing daily.

♦ The psychostimulants (Ritalin, Dexedrine and Cylert) are the most effective medications for ADD.

♦ Dexedrine may be effective when Ritalin is not and vice-versa.

♦ Cylert is occasionally effective (2% of the time) if Ritalin and Dexedrine are not.

♦ Ritalin and Dexedrine tablets treat discreet four-hour segments of life, while Ritalin SR and Dexedrine Spansules may be effective for considerably longer periods of time.

♦ The amount of medication is dictated by clinical response.

♦ There is little correlation between dose and weight.

♦ There is little correlation between effective dose and the severity of ADD.

- If no effect is noted, not enough medication is being prescribed, or it is not being taken.

- Avoid the *drug holiday* concept.

- Use of medication is dependent upon the child's need, taking social interaction as well as academic performance into account.

- Medication will help the child with ADD become more responsive to behavior management interventions and to his academic program.

- The child must be held accountable for oppositional defiant behavior over which the psychostimulants have little, if any, control.

- The psychostimulants, when used appropriately, are remarkably safe and, if diagnosis is correct, remarkably effective.

- Other medications include the tricyclic antidepressants (TCA's), imipramine (Tofranil), and desipramine (Norpramiń). They should be used only if side effects preclude the use of psychostimulants or if a significant co-morbidity such as anxiety or depression exists.

- Clonidine, which is not particularly effective for ADD, may alleviate out-of-control rage outbursts (dyscontrol) which may co-exist with ADD. It can be used in conjunction with the psychostimulants. It lowers the incidence of tics and enables the use of lower doses of stimulant medication.

- Medication should be a concomitant therapy and not a last resort if all else fails.

Behavior Management

Medication is beneficial for most children with attention deficit disorder. Behavior management is necessary for all. You notice I say *behavior management*, not modification. If we get wrapped up in the word *modification*, we may really begin to believe we can actually modify someone's behavior, and we are going to anticipate permanent results from our efforts by next week. That just does not happen. Remember what I said previously. It is the parent's and teacher's job to act as a governor for the disinhibition these children experience. They provide the brakes to inappropriate behaviors. They must make the child aware of socially unacceptable behavior, and they must do so over and over again, year after year, for when they withdraw their surveillance and intervention, it is likely that the child will return to his inattentive, impulsive state.

In directing our attention to behavior, we must constantly keep in mind the distinction between *incompetent behavior* due to the attention deficit disorder, and *oppositional defiant behavior* over which, we have to believe, the child can gain control. Incompetent, skill-deficit ADD behaviors are not to be punished, but they must receive our attention and intervention. When the child is noncompliant and behaves in an unacceptable oppositional way, he should be disciplined in the true sense of the word, *i.e.*, *taught by consequence*, and given assistance and cognitive cues to develop self-control over time. Behavior can be managed only in proportion to the child's recognition of the consequence of his actions and in response to what he is specifically taught. In managing behaviors, it is important to manage one's own. Out-of-control parent behavior exacerbates the inappropriate behavior of children. Logical, predictable consequences are far more effective than lectures, nagging or coercion.

Dr. Tom Phelan's *1,2,3 Magic System* of behavior management is highly recommended for young children (see Appendix B). This is an excellent program. Dr. Phelan implores us to train, not persuade, and points out that young children are not little adults. According to him, "Young children are selfish, impulsive, undisciplined and irrational." Thus, it is imperative that we not try to reason with them. Do not ever get involved in lengthy explanations as to why the child should comply with requests. In his booklet, Dr. Phelan urges parents: "Don't show your emotions, don't get angry and don't talk." "Act, don't yak." He is an excellent child psychologist who may have such a good understanding of attention deficit disorder because he has a son with the condition.

To stop inappropriate action, Dr. Phelan uses a time-out method and, to start action, employs positive reinforcement such as a token system. The nature of token systems must be changed frequently to keep the ADD youngster interested. Children with attention deficit disorder benefit from immediate consequences and have a very hard time waiting for later reward. To take advantage of this characteristic, some suggest giving the youngster all his tokens or all of his rewards at one time, then taking away tokens as a result of noncompliance with the rules. This method is called *response cost*. One must be careful with response-cost methods, however, for many children respond by giving up instead of becoming more motivated.

A reward system I like is the use of a grab bag. Write on slips of paper a variety of different rewards, some pretty substantial and others relatively minor. Going to the store to get a candy bar, a toy model or another video game, or going to the park, ice skating rink or sledding are examples. The child is allowed to remove one of these slips from the bag when he has complied with the contract you've established. While this is effective for most, other children will be more motivated by specific knowledge of the goal.

Always remember to label verbal rewards. When the child complies with a request such as picking up his coat, don't just say "thanks," but "Thank you for picking up your coat." Let him always know the deed for which you are thanking him.

In attempting to obtain compliance with requests, make certain the child understands perfectly what you've requested of him. Often the hyperactive child zooming by doesn't have the vaguest notion of what you have asked of him. After issuing a command or request, it is a good idea to ask the child what it is you said. If he can parrot it back to you, you know that it's in his computer. Then, if he doesn't comply, you have grounds for negative consequences. If you don't know what's in his computer, you really have no justification for punishment.

Avoid chain commands. Give him one thing to do and see that he does it. Verbally reward him for his accomplishment, then give him another task. Don't string together three or four requests at one time such as, "Pick up your boots you left in the hall, put your coat in the closet, take out the trash and feed the dog." All he will hear is *dog*. He will end up playing with Fido while his boots, coat and the trash go unattended.

Don't be vague. The one I really like is "act your age." Often my medical students don't know how a three-year-old or a five-year-old acts. Yet we're expecting a young child to both know and to act in accordance with the norm of a child of a given chronological age, with certain cognitive efficiencies and physical prowess. Clearly tell the child what you want of him and expect it to be accomplished.

To illustrate how to distinguish skill-deficit ADD incompetent behaviors due to attention deficit disorder from oppositional noncompliant behaviors, I like to use the following example: The child comes in and puts his feet up on the couch. You say "Robert, take your feet off the couch." Robert immediately takes his feet off the couch. He has complied. Then it's a good idea to say, "Thank you for taking your feet off the couch." A few minutes later he again has his feet on the couch. You again tell him to take his feet off the couch. Don't get angry and don't punish him, for you are acting as his governor in helping to make up for a skill deficit. He immediately takes his feet off the couch; he has again complied with your request. He may do it again. It is perfectly all right to remind him that this is now the third time you have made this request, but again no punishment.

Contrast this with noncompliant behavior. You say, "Robert, take your feet off the couch," and he goes on reading his comic book. That's noncompliance. He should receive negative consequences. Even worse and obviously oppositional, when you say "Robert, take your feet off the couch," he mouths off in a loud voice, "I don't have to take my feet off the couch—they're not dirty. You're always bitching at me." He should experience immediate negative consequences for this noncompliant, defiant behavior.

Consequences are so important! . . . that is, after the neurological basis of the disorder has been addressed. Impulsivity, overactivity, inappropriate social responding and negative behavior are markedly impervious to the effects of consequences *before* medical intervention. Once a medication regime has been established, predictable consequences, administered within a framework of a structure, and logic are crucial. The child is then able to learn that when he intentionally breaks a toy, he doesn't get another. If he abuses his puppy, he loses the puppy for a period of time. If he leaves his bicycle in the yard and it is stolen, he doesn't get another one, at least not until Christmas.

Cognitive behavior management is an attempt to bring behavior management *inside* the child. It is internal locus of control. It is an attempt to supplant our external efforts at governing the situation. In essence it is moving from autocracy to democracy and including the child in the decision-making process. Methods include visual cueing, audiotaped reminders and written self-instruction. Much has been written about it. There is considerable question, however, regarding its effectiveness with the child with ADD who usually cognitively understands how he is supposed to behave, but who cannot respond appropriately because of his impulsivity.

The importance of appropriate referral to a child psychiatrist for the management of anxiety and depression with or without ADD has been previously mentioned. This is to be encouraged, particularly when treatment involves nonstimulant psychopharmacology. Align yourself with a competent, compatible psychiatrist and also align yourself with one or more child psychologists. Be quick to refer to a child psychologist the child with significant oppositional defiant behavior, for if intervention is not effective, conduct disorder results. You can build a rewarding relationship with *your psychologist* as you become *his physician.* You prescribe and monitor medication as he attempts to probe more deeply the roots of family dysfunction and evolve an effective behavior management plan for those children for whom you do not feel comfortable providing their total care.

◆ ◆ ◆ ◆ ◆ ◆

BEHAVIOR MANAGEMENT

◆ Incompetent ADD skill-deficit behaviors are not to be punished.

◆ Time out is an effective way to extinguish unwanted behavior.

◆ A positive reward system helps initiate desirable behavior.

◆ Control by consequences, not by reasoning.

◆ Don't yell, argue or hit. "Act, don't yak."

◆ Label the verbal rewards.

◆ Avoid chain commands.

◆ Cognitive behavior management is usually ineffective without considerable long-term training of the child.

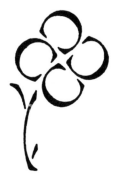

Responsibility Training

I cannot stress enough the importance of responsibility training. It is often neglected. It should be an integral part of the care of children with ADD. These children must be taught how to work. It is important that they develop a good work ethic, for, in all probability, they will have to work twice as hard as the next fellow to be successful. Don't feel too sorry for them because of this, for work properly done can be a pleasurable and rewarding experience, vastly enhancing the child's self esteem. Remember grandmother's rule: "Work first, play later." Saturday morning is housecleaning time. You help with the housecleaning and then you can go out to play ball. You get your work done first, then you have an opportunity to play as a reward.

It is important that there be a contractual arrangement, hopefully consistent, between home and school. House rules should be explicit and obeyed. The child should have regular daily chores to do at home and should become the teacher's helper in school.

Children with ADD need help with organization—a place for their socks, a place for their shirts—and they should put the toothpaste away with the cap on. Children with ADD should all have a watch and learn to organize time. See to it that the child with ADD wears her watch and that you often ask her how much time before such-and-such happens. A non-digital watch is better for the ADD child, for he can see time as a wholistic concept. Digital watches are too much like his personality style and reinforce *blips* of activity rather than an organized whole. An organization calendar will help ADD children look at their lives. Structure is important. They need a specific time for meals, a specific time for bed and a specific time to get up in the morning. I will mention this to some parents and the mother might shrug and say, "We just don't have a very structured family." If that doesn't change, they are going to have a totally unstructured child who is not going to benefit from goodness of fit, for goodness of fit for children with ADD requires structure, at least to the best of the parent's ability.

One of our most important jobs as parents is to educate our children for separation. Thought must be given to this soon after birth, for it is early in life that we begin to instill in our children those qualities which allow separation from us to be comfortable and rewarding. We may foster dependency to satisfy our own needs to be considered worthwhile, but more often it is because we are afraid to let go of our unfinished products.

Excellent responsibility programs for children beginning at age three are available (see Appendix B). Children at three should begin to be taught responsibility—all children, not just children with attention deficit disorder. In children with ADD it is imperative. Children should be making their beds and keeping their rooms clean. The sobering statistic that 22 million adult children in this country have returned home to live with their parents should encourage parents to teach their children the value of work and responsibility. "Indulge now, pay later." You pay, but the child pays more dearly.

◆ ◆ ◆ ◆ ◆ ◆

RESPONSIBILITY TRAINING

- Work first, play later.

- Home chores.

- Teacher's helper.

- Educate for separation.

- Teach organization.

- Indulge now, pay later.

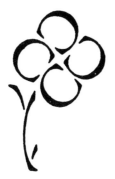

Self-Image Enhancement

Self-image enhancement must receive priority in the care of the ADD child. It is crucial that the child feel good about himself even though he has a disability. We want a child who can establish lasting interpersonal relationships, and that can only occur in the presence of love of self.

Parents must expect good performance. If there are no expectations, they have emotionally abandoned their child. It is important that they not exaggerate by rewarding a child for something that he should be expected to do considering his age and intellectual capacity. So often a mother or teacher is surprised at a particular performance and will go on and on about how great the child is for having done something one would really expect of the child. It's understandable that, if he has never done it before, it is going to deserve some comment, but help parents not to go overboard. It will erode self image if they think the commonplace is so great. Just a labeled verbal reward, such as "Thank you for taking out the garbage," should suffice. Certainly encourage them not to say something like, "You took out the garbage. I can't believe it. It's the first time you've done that in weeks!" Parents should not bring up prior failures and indiscretions, particularly at a time when some good has just been accomplished.

The following are other suggestions to share with parents of ADD children.

Contributing to the family—If the child contributes, the child feels better about himself. See to it that he does his chores. Don't blame, don't shame and don't humiliate. Don't say, "You keep that up and you won't amount to anything."

Realistic expectations—Always start with a task that can be successfully completed, then work up from there. If he has a major behavior problem and you can expect him realistically to behave for no longer than five minutes of free play, let him out for five minutes, watch him carefully and praise him for his good behavior during that period of time. You've got to see that he succeeds. Mel Levine, M.D., calls constant lack of success "*success deprivation.*" Nothing erodes self image more than this. Praise and encouraging words are important, but they are of little value when compared to succeeding.

Consistency—You must be consistent in your management, especially as it relates to discipline, for inconsistency leads to considerable anxiety. Much of the anxiety in children in dysfunctional families comes from inconsistency. An extreme example is physical abuse one minute and telling the child how much you love him the next. The child may be better off in a consistent, mildly abusing environment than one that fluctuates between affection and exorbitant punishment.

Affirmations—Affirmations are of unparalleled importance. We become so accustomed to talking about time out. Let's think of affirmations as *time in*: "Your needs are important to me." "I'll always love you (unconditional love)." "It's ok to be angry." "You belong here." Even with negative behavior, a parent can be affirming: "You are too neat a kid to act like that." "It's not like you and I won't have it." Children who receive affirmations are more secure and feel better about themselves even though they are having a tough time doing their math or sitting still in English class.

Physical appearance—Physical appearance and grooming

are important. Attention should be given to weight reduction if indicated, and enuresis should be treated. There is no causal correlation between nocturnal enuresis and ADD. However, they may, and do, co-exist. Stimulant medications appear to alert *all* the attention centers, including attention to body signals, and thus may help some children overcome enuresis.

Nurture skills—Evident skills must be nurtured such as ability in art, music or karate. These children often have good rhythm, though they may have difficulty reading music. Sports may be important. Participation should be encouraged but the child should not be pushed unless he is capable of accomplishment. Children with ADD, particularly those with hyperactivity, tend toward the extremes of motor coordination and athletic ability. A disproportionately large number are athletically talented and excel in a variety of sports, while others display significant visual-motor problems which interfere with sports such as baseball and basketball. Sports such as swimming, track and wrestling generally can be accomplished without much difficulty even in children who have some visual-motor perceptual deficits or difficulties in fine-motor control. These are gross-motor activities requiring strength and endurance, which the ADD child may have in abundance. These sports also do not require intense interpersonal relationships, a common requirement of team sports. Karate is a great activity for youngsters with attention deficit disorder, for it not only is an enjoyable sport but it teaches discipline, as well as respect, and it rewards effort. Working for concrete objectives, such as belts, can focus the ADD child's energies. Medication can aid sports accomplishments and team cooperation significantly.

Adaptive P.E. programs—If the child has particular problems with gross- motor efficiency, an adaptive physical education program may be indicated. You do not want to set this child up for failure. If he is somewhat clumsy and slow, you should not insist upon competition with a more physically competent peer group.

Avoid threats—Never threaten abandonment, mutilation or homicide. "You do that once more and I'm stopping the car and leaving you by the side of the road." "Shape up or I'll pull your fingers out one by one." "I'll kill you if you do that." In my day we were threatened with being sent to the orphanage. Don't use threats, for in so doing you both create subtle anxiety in the child and lose his respect. You gain respect and the ability to influence behavior by making the rules clear and then insisting upon compliance.

Medication—Medication often helps others to look at the child with attention deficit disorder more favorably. In many cases it helps improve peer relationships and lessen rejection.

Avoid "how comes?"—Now that you understand the condition, avoid the demeaning *how comes*? "How come you can remember what Uncle Joe had to eat at the church picnic three years ago and you can't remember what I just told you?" "How come you can't do it? You could do it yesterday." "How come you spend so much time on all that detail and you don't know what the big picture is all about?" "How come you are climbing the walls in school? You do just fine in my office, so I know you can do it." Sooner or later the child will begin to wonder "how come?" and think of himself as deficient or stupid. This may lead to acting-out behavior, for we all know that "It's better to be a jerk than to be stupid." Or the child will feel demeaned and withdraw for self-preservation.

♦ ♦ ♦ ♦ ♦ ♦

SELF-IMAGE ENHANCEMENT

♦ Expect performance.

♦ Don't blame, don't shame, don't humiliate.

♦ Always start with a task that can be successfully accomplished.

♦ Avoid inconsistency.

♦ Affirmations are important.

♦ Nurture evident skills.

♦ Never threaten unrealistic punishment—in fact, never threaten anything.

♦ Medication helps others to look upon the child more favorably.

♦ Avoid the "how comes?".

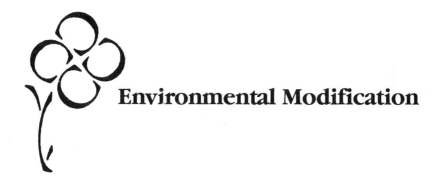

Environmental Modification

Environmental modification is another facet of the multimodal approach to treatment. To be truly effective, one must first find the child's best environment. Some ADD children perform best in a quiet, low-distraction situation while others will actually perform better with music playing. In school it is usually best for children to have separate desks for independent work and for them to be away from distractions such as the window or the air conditioner. Being near the teacher may help some, while others perform best when surrounded by hard-working students.

If distractibility were the whole story, the ADD child would be expected to perform best in a monotonous, sterile environment, but such is not the case. Such an environment is too boring. The child with ADD requires a little distraction just to fan the fire and keep things warmed up enough to provide the energy necessary to sustain attention. It is perhaps best, though, that distracting mobiles not be hung from the ceiling obstructing the line of vision to the teacher. If possible, provide all children in the class with a quiet space such as a cubicle into which they can voluntarily escape classroom distraction when they feel it will enhance study efforts. Soft sponge ear plugs are, at times, of considerable benefit should the child choose to use them to reduce the effect of classroom noise. Such assistance is especially helpful for tests and prolonged independent seat work.

At home consideration should also be given to work environment preference. Does he perform better in bright or subdued light? Is absolute quiet or background music more facilitating? Does he prefer a warm environment or does he like it cool? These preferences will influence performance. Work periods should be short, routine should be consistent, and allowance should be made for some physical movement.

A punching bag or pillow can be utilized for moments of frustration and aggression. Do your best to provide the child a place for safe, free play. Let his room be his castle as far as decor is concerned, but see to it that he keeps it neat.

◆ ◆ ◆ ◆ ◆ ◆

ENVIRONMENTAL MODIFICATIONS

- ◆ Place student in the place determined to be most effective for learning.

- ◆ Place away from major distractions.

- ◆ Provide a quiet place to study.

- ◆ Don't make environment too boring.

- ◆ Consider the child's work environment preference.

- ◆ Make work periods short.

- ◆ Plan activities which encourage brief periods of physical movement.

Social Skills Training

Children with attention deficit disorder are often bossy and boastful. Many have difficulty making friends. Social skills training may be of help, but it's unlikely that a separate course in social skills will be of much benefit. While there is usually good performance during the sessions, carryover effects have been difficult to demonstrate. Daily reminders by teachers and parents regarding socially accepted behavior and establishing specific social goals which are reinforced are of much greater value. Teach manners. Generally the more socially adept the child is, the more accepted he is. It is interesting to observe children with ADD when you suggest eye contact. They may stare right through you. Eye contact should be encouraged when giving the child positive feedback or specific directions. Demanding eye contact when giving negative messages can demean a child and make him angry. Forced eye contact is rarely helpful.

Appearance was addressed previously in *maintaining a good self-image*. This is part of social skills training as well. Parents must help their child present himself to his society, particularly his peer group, in as acceptable a way as possible. Sometimes that is tie-dyed jeans, untied shoes and a ponytail. For other peer groups, "preppy" is in.

Teaching boundaries is also helpful. You must help both parents and child understand people's need for space and that the child should not invade another's physical space unless invited to do so. Did you ever watch a child with ADD go bounding down the hall in school with his arms flailing about? He often inadvertently creates strife. It is not a bad idea to teach the youngster to keep his hands in his pockets in the hall. Try to help him to be aware that people do not like his tugging on them.

◆ ◆ ◆ ◆ ◆ ◆

SOCIAL SKILLS TRAINING

◆   Structured social skills training sessions have been found to be of little value because of the lack of generalization.

◆   Be aware of the importance of eye contact and when it is useful.

◆   Teach manners.

◆   Neat, cared-for appearance is important as long as it is in keeping with peer-group acceptance.

◆   Help him not to invade another's space.

◆   Help the child understand inappropriate social behaviors and learn more appropriate means of meeting his attentional needs.

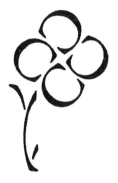

School Program

The school must assume its vital role. For treatment to be successful, the child's academic environment must be changed, work segments shortened, lesson plans modified and demands on the child's abilities kept within the parameters of his skill. For years many have felt that ADD is an exceptional educational need (EEN), and should be declared such under law. In September, 1991, a memo from the United States Department of Education gave sanction to including ADD under the "Other Health Impaired" category for the purpose of establishing eligibility for special educational consideration in compliance with P.L. 94-142, *i.e.,* Public Law No. 142 of the 94th Congress, the Education of the Handicapped Act (EHA), now called the *Individuals with Disabilities Education Act, (IDEA).* This law guarantees a free appropriate public school education (FAPE) to all children regardless of disability. An excerpt from the U. S. Department of Education Memo is included in Appendix K.

All children under the law are to be educated in the least restrictive environment (LRE). Generally children with attention deficit disorder should receive a modified academic program in the regular classroom.   They should be placed in special education self-contained classrooms only if other concomitant deficiencies such as severe learning disabilities, mental retardation, or severe behavior disorders dictate that such special educational assistance would be in the best interests of the child.

Teachers must anticipate and prepare. They must prepare for the presence of the child with ADD in the classroom. They can do so only by having received the academic and medical records prior to the first day of school. Learning deficiencies should be made known to the teacher, for the teacher must fully understand the child's academic strengths and weaknesses. The teacher must be aware of medication employed, dose and time of administration, possible side effects and anticipated benefits.

The teacher must anticipate and prepare for transitions, for most ADD children will have difficulty with transitions, whether from room to room, from playground back to classroom, or from teacher to teacher. The child must be assisted ahead of time with transitions. It is not a bad idea for the teacher to meet the child with attention deficit disorder at the door as he comes in from recess, place a reassuring touch on his arm and remind him of the behavior expected in the classroom. Children with attention deficit disorder, if they are relatively free of oppositional behaviors, very much wish to behave.

The child with ADD is troubled by the same *lethal cluster* that impedes the progress of the LD student:

1. *Fitting work into time.* Time is too short to get the answers down on paper or it's too long a time until the deadline for completion of the assignment. "Your paper on the rain forest will be due a week from Monday."

2. *Written output.* "Can't I just tell you or show you what it's about?"

3. *Tests (measures of mastery).* Test anxiety is almost as prevalent in the child with ADD as in the learning disabled. Alice Koontz tells us that to a youngster with LD, a test by another name (*exam* or *quiz*) is still a four-letter word.

The classroom teacher should have available relatively immediate consultation from the school psychologist. The school psychologist must serve as a resource consultant to the classroom teacher regarding behavior. It is the school psychologist who should have the necessary knowledge to deal most effectively with significant behavior problems as they arise.

I advise that children with ADD and/or LD have regular daily study hours at home beginning in second or third grade. For example, thirty minutes four to five days a week. The child gets to choose whether the study time is after school or after supper, but, once the choice is made that time is it for one month. The teacher is to indicate material for home study. As the child gets older and the work becomes more difficult, the study periods should be lengthened to approximately one to two hours a day, five days a week, of mandatory home study. In college the average should be two hours of study for each classroom hour.

A behavior management system should be in place which is as consistent as possible between home and school. The cooperation of the parents must be elicited, fully realizing that such cooperation may be spotty, or, at times nonexistent.

It's a good idea to teach youngsters with ADD computer keyboarding skills early in the elementary grades, for the computer is going to be a godsend in their educational program. The computer is tailor-made for a child with attention deficit disorder. The immediate feedback is very beneficial to the child who has problems attending. The computer can help the disorganized child organize his thoughts and develop plans for task accomplishment. Unfortunately, in some schools, the child who is not doing well because of his attention deficit disorder and perhaps some learning problems, does not have access to the computer, for the computer is held out as a reward for academic achievement. This seems kind of backwards to me. Also, in embracing technology, we must not overlook the teacher's human embrace, for touching is so important to these children. *Hug therapy* is perhaps as important as *computer therapy* and behavior management. (See Appendix O for a wonderful handout for parents on hugging.)

It is quite probable that by the end of this decade computer technology will be the basic educational tool for children with ADD. This stands to reason, for the computer sustains the child's attention. It is like having a personal teacher who provides material in an interesting way (graphics) and gives immediate reinforcement. Through the computer there is constant adjustment to rate of learning, and it can capture the imagination of the child as it encourages the ADD student on to greater success. We will be hearing more and more about computer educational systems (CES) and computer-assisted education.

Children with ADD have difficulty with auditory memory as well as attention. They often miss portions of the teacher's verbal instructions. An inexpensive tape recorder can allow the child the opportunity to return to instructions again and again. However, incorporating multisensory strategies into the learning process more effectively meets the needs of children who are not strong auditory learners, as well as those who are.

Frequent contact between parents and teachers is imperative. It is my general recommendation that no more than two weeks go by without some type of contact between the teacher and the parents of a youngster with attention deficit disorder. What must be avoided is waiting six weeks for a parent/teacher conference and then unloading upon parents failures, indiscretions, and misbehaviors for the whole grading period. Waiting a long time for grades renders them relatively ineffective. A child with attention deficit disorder needs a report on how he is doing almost daily.

Helping to organize the child for school is essential. One of the most effective tools I have seen is *The Organization Notebook for Class and Homework* (see Appendix B). The *notebook* is a 3-ring binder which comes with (1) a weekly "Homework Assignment" sheet to be changed each week; (2) pocket folders large enough to put papers in easily and color coded for quick reference; and (3) directions for organizing the forgetful, disorganized student, as well as a plan for close monitoring between parent and teacher when needed.

Children with ADD typically have grades all over the map. I recently reviewed the report card of a youngster who had *A, B, C, D* and *F*. The *A* was in social studies, not physical education. When the subject interests them, they often become absorbed to the detriment of less interesting work. There is only so much energy, so effort will be expended where success appears most possible. Some teachers provide a better fit. The child's social studies' teacher, because of tolerance and understanding of ADD, may have provided the child a better fit than the English teacher, in whose class he made a D.

There must be sensitive handling of medications in school without shaming the child. I've heard of occasions in which a loudspeaker announcement directed Billy to go to the office to get his behavior pill. Be ever so careful not to embarrass these children. It is easy for most of us to make an unthinking comment unless we give conscious attention to the deleterious effect of such action. You must help educate the teacher and school on their responsibilities to administer medication, document its administration, and notify you of both benefits and side effects.

In attending to the classroom needs of the ADD child, we may experience something of a renaissance in education. So many adaptations favorable to the education of the child with ADD benefit all children. We might begin by eliminating competition in early grades, emphasizing cooperation instead. Hopefully there will be a renewed interest in quality of work rather than quantity. The quantity required should be dictated by the child's learning needs and not by a particular curriculum or unit requirement mandated by the state. It is likely that in the future most schools' first four educational years will be ungraded (K-3). The appreciation that all persons, including the teacher, have strengths and weaknesses will be stressed. A true concept of fairness may evolve, not a concept which says if we do it for one we have to do it for all, but rather an understanding which directs us to provide according to need.

As a teacher provides the stimuli to sustain the attention of the child with ADD, he or she will find that the entire class is showing renewed interest. The teacher will move about the room, change the tone and volume of her voice, act out salient points, always summarize the lesson and inject humor into the classroom. Instruction in the organization of work will take place, and there will be increased positive reinforcement with no humiliation.

Because of the profound necessity for involvement of both medicine and education, attention deficit disorder may well serve as the catalyst to break down the artificial barriers that presently exist between the two professions.

♦ ♦ ♦ ♦ ♦ ♦

SCHOOL PROGRAM

♦ The school has a vital role in treatment of ADD.

♦ ADD has been recognized as a disability by the Federal Department of Education (DOE).

♦ Most children with ADD can and should be taught in the regular classroom.

♦ Adaptations and modifications should be made in keeping with both the child's disabilities and his abilities.

♦ Home study hours are important.

♦ The behavior management system should be consistent between home and school.

♦ Computers will play an increasingly important role in the education of the child with ADD.

♦ Frequent contact between parents and teachers is imperative.

♦ Changes in educational requirements and teaching methods to meet the needs of the child with ADD will benefit all children.

♦ *Fair* doesn't mean if you do it for one you do it for all. Rather, true fairness means providing according to need.

Attend to the
Co-Morbidities

We will not be successful in our treatment unless we attend to the *co-morbidities*, those conditions that may co-exist with ADD. The child with severe defiant noncompliant behavior may require a school placement with segregated resource instruction for the behaviorally disturbed (BD), or the emotionally disturbed (ED). He often requires the intervention of a child psychologist as well.

The learning disabled child must receive appropriate learning disability assistance. While classwork in a resource room may be necessary, children with learning differences and behavioral difficulties must be allowed to participate in regular school activities as much as possible.

Occupational therapy assistance may be of benefit. The occupational therapist can help the teacher by suggesting equipment and methods to help the child compensate for fine-motor inefficiency and visual-motor and motor-planning deficits.

We must watch for evidence of depression, particularly in teenage girls, and treat it as a separate entity. It may be a co-morbidity with attention deficit disorder. It is not an inevitable consequence. The same holds true for anxiety, which can be a co-morbidity, especially if there is a dysfunctional family which happens to have a child with attention deficit disorder. To deal effectively with depression and anxiety, referral to a child psychiatrist will usually be in your young patient's best interest. The co-morbidities, rather than ADD, often determine outcome as much or more than the ADD. Generally, undesirable outcome is a result of poor management of the ADD, the presence of oppositional defiant disorder inappropriately treated, or the presence of a genetically-based conduct disorder.

◆ ◆ ◆ ◆ ◆ ◆

ATTEND TO THE CO-MORBIDITIES

♦   Oppositional defiant behavior disorder (ODD).

♦   Learning disabilities (LD).

♦   Fine- and gross-motor deficits.

♦   Depression.

♦   Anxiety.

♦   Refer to a child psychiatrist or psychologist.

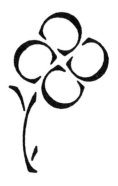

Attend to Family Problems

The family is vital to the positive development of the ADD child. We need to attend to the co-morbidities of the child, but often before that we need to attend to family problems, particularly marital discord, which can have its origin in attempting to parent a child with attention deficit disorder. Often there is polarization, especially with regard to different disciplinary styles and the question of indulgence. A child with attention deficit disorder can, indeed, create a chaotic family. We find that, once parents begin to understand attention deficit disorder, their differences often decrease. This is particularly true as a spouse also recognizes residuals of the disorder in the mate. If the parents are reasonably secure individuals, once there is understanding, tolerance usually follows. Involvement in support groups is immeasurably beneficial in this process.

Insecurity poses a problem, especially as it relates to depression in a parent. It is hard to be consistent and sure of one's decisions when one is depressed. The person who is depressed has a tendency to blame others for her sadness. Depression does not fit well with attention deficit disorder. A depressed parent often inter-prets the incompetent behaviors of the child or spouse as intentional malice and personal affront. Encourage the depressed parent to seek treatment. There are many medications now available that significantly alter the symptoms of depression. To be most effective, medication should be accompanied by counseling or psychotherapy.

Alcohol or drug abuse is especially devastating. Each results in a dysfunctional family which has a terrible time being consistent. To benefit the child, this dependency disorder should be treated. We must not forget the detrimental effects of the co-dependency role. Whether or not an alcoholic parent does or does not seek treatment, it is helpful to recommend ALANON or a similar program to the spouse.

In addressing family problems, it is important to consider residual ADD. As I mentioned previously, 30% of fathers and 20% of mothers of children with attention deficit disorder are believed to have characteristics of the disorder. If it is present, it is important to share this awareness with the child and spouse and all work together, with the help of a knowledgeable professional.

Attend to the co-morbidities, attend to family problems, and encourage involvement in a support group for parents of children and adolescents with ADD. I consider attendance at support group meetings a critical part of treatment. CH.A.D.D., *Children With Attention Deficit Disorders*, and ADDA, *Attention Deficit Disorder Association*, are the national support groups with chapters in many cities throughout the country (Appendix P). Other helpful support groups which offer assistance for some of the co-morbidities associated with ADD are also listed in Appendix P. A support group provides not only support and education for parents, but an opportunity for parents and professionals to share their experiences. As professionals, we learn much from the experience of parents. Parents learn from and accept a tremendous amount of help from each other.

◆ ◆ ◆ ◆ ◆ ◆

ATTEND TO FAMILY PROBLEMS

♦ Marital discord.

♦ Depression.

♦ Alcohol or drug abuse.

♦ Residual ADD in a parent.

♦ Attend support group meetings.

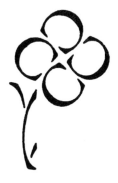

What Won't Work

As we approach the end of this book, let's consider what doesn't work in the treatment of attention deficit disorder. Restriction of sugar, food coloring or preservatives won't solve the problem. Desensitizing to molds, treating real or imagined yeast infections or subjecting the child to spinal adjustments won't alleviate ADD. Counseling of young children does not work. The characteristics of attention deficit disorder preclude success. Counseling can help solve family problems, and adolescents and young adults often benefit from counseling to resolve the emotional effects of long-standing attention disorders. Counseling is only helpful if the child finds value in the activity and wishes to participate.

Psychotherapy, by itself, is of little value in treating attention deficit disorder. It can, at best, help the child become comfortable with her failures. It does not help the deficit in sustained attention, impulsivity or hyperactivity caused by a biologic abnormality. Play therapy, *i.e.*, psychotherapy for the younger child, is, likewise, of little benefit as a single treatment of attention deficit disorder. Psychotherapy may be of distinct benefit in resolving family problems and dealing with certain co-morbidities.

Physical punishment must be avoided. Children with attention deficit disorder have a tendency to be somewhat aggressive, particularly if they develop defiant behaviors. Those children physically punished will model the aggression and hit others, particularly children younger than themselves. Even when children comply momentarily because of physical punishment, the residual humiliation and anger they experience lead to long-term social and emotional overlays that can be exceedingly counterproductive.

Attempts at improving moral control by strict religious dictum will not help, although the presence of religious value structures within the family is often beneficial. Blame, shame, or humiliation only make the child feel worse about something he cannot control.

♦ ♦ ♦ ♦ ♦ ♦

WHAT WON'T WORK

- ♦ Restriction of sugar, food colorings, yeast

- ♦ Counseling or psychotherapy alone

- ♦ Physical punishment

- ♦ Religious dictum

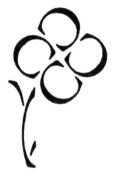

Conclusion

Goodness of fit is the key to the appropriate treatment of the child with attention deficit disorder. Understanding by you, parents and teachers improves the goodness of fit. We all become more tolerant. Medication can almost normalize the child's impulsive, inattentive behavior so that he conforms better and is more accepted by his peer group, his family and his teachers. Giving him frequent, repetitive feedback and encouragement improves the fit. He is then able to sustain attention for a period of time until the next reminder comes his way. Emphasizing quality, not quantity, improves goodness of fit. It affords the child an opportunity to have pride of accomplishment while avoiding negative consequences in response to messy, hastily done, inaccurate work. Attending to the co-morbidities, family problems and the child's appearance helps his chances for success.

Several years ago my friend Eric Denhoff gave me what he called his short course on attention deficit disorder. He described the child with ADD as one who "never sits, never listens, never completes and never succeeds."

By improving the goodness of fit, you enhance the child's ability to be competent, productive and fulfilled. The future quality of the ADD child's life will be determined one success at a time. As his attending physician, *you* can make a difference. You can set in motion the changes which will dramatically and positively alter his life.

IN SUMMARY

♦   Attention is the basic neurologic function.

♦   There can be no education without attention.

♦   Attention Deficit Disorder is a biologic abnormality of the nervous system. It is not due to poor parenting or poor teaching.

♦   Characteristics of attention deficit disorder include:

  • Episodic inattention.

  • Impulsivity.

  • Hyperactivity or activity-level problems.

♦   It is a definite disability identified specifically for inclusion under P.L. 94-142 (Education of the Handicapped Act) and Section 504 of P.L. 93-112.

♦   There is no specific test for attention deficit disorder. Diagnosis is based upon observations of parents and teachers, accompanied by psychological and educational test data. Physicians and mental health professionals interpret the data and exclude other disorders which can affect attention.

♦ Therapy is multimodal consisting of:

- Education of parents, teachers, and the child.

- Medication, which is remarkably safe and very effective.

- Application of adaptive academic programs and behavior management.

♦ Undesirable outcome is most often dependent upon the presence of a conduct disorder, which may or may not have its origin in oppositional defiant behavior. Oppositional defiant behavior disorder (ODD) is not attention deficit disorder (ADD), but it is a frequent co-morbidity, especially when the ADD child is punished for behavior over which he has little control, or receives excessive negative feedback.

♦ Skill training *per se* is relatively ineffective because the skills do not usually generalize outside the therapy situation. The child with ADD cognitively knows what to do, he just can't do it. However, attention to social skills in daily life is a critical part of the behavioral intervention program.

♦ The goal of therapy is to improve the goodness of fit between the child with ADD and his environment.

♦ Our job, as the attending physician, is to protect the child against his own vulner-abilities until his skills increase.

♦ ♦ ♦ ♦ ♦ ♦

To understand ADD is to diagnose it. To understand ADD is to treat it. I hope that this book, in some measure, has helped you better understand your young patient with attention deficit disorder. If so, he and his parents will be grateful. You, in return, will have become a more complete physician.

Thank you for your attention.

Stephen Copps, M.D.

APPENDICES

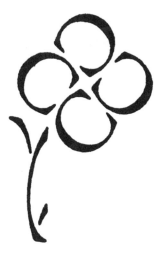

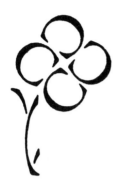

Appendices

APPENDIX A

NEUROPHYSIOLOGY OF ATTENTION
DEFICIT DISORDER

Review Articles

1. Calis, K.A., Grothe, D.R., & Elia, J. (1990). Therapy reviews: Attention-deficit hyperactivity disorder. *Clinical Pharmacology,* *9,* 632-642.

2. Hunt, R.D., Mandel, L., Lau, S., & Hughes, M. (1991). Neurological Theories of ADHD and Ritalin, in L. L. Greenhill and B. B. Osman (Eds.), *Ritalin Theory and Patient Management.* New York: Mary Ann Liebert, Inc. Publishers.

3. Zametkin, A.J., & Borcherding, B.G. (1989). The neuropharmacology of attention-deficit hyperactivity disorder. *Annual Review of Medicine, 40,* 447-451.

APPENDIX B

EQUIP YOUR PRACTICE FOR THE CARE
OF THE CHILD WITH ADD

You have completed a primer on ADD. Now more fully equip yourself for the task at hand by reading cover to cover Barkley's book on attention deficit disorder.

Attention Deficit Hyperactivity Disorder: A Handbook for Diagnosis and Treatment. Russell A. Barkley, Guilford Publications, Inc., Dept. 4W, 72 Spring Street, New York, New York 10012, (800) 365-7006 (747 pages hardcover).

Add to your patient pamphlet rack a simple booklet on ADD.

About Attention Deficit Disorder, A Scriptographic Book by Channing L. Bete Co., South Deerfield, Massachusetts 01373, (800) 628-7733. Request booklet No. 48935 (15 pages paper cover).

To keep up to date as painlessly as possible, order the printed proceedings from the annual CH.A.D.D. conference and plan on doing this every year.

Order from: C.A.S.E.T. Associates, 3927 Old Lee Highway, Fairfax, Virginia 22030, (703) 352-0091. Proceedings of the 1991 CH.A.D.D. Conference. This company has available audiotapes of all presentations at the 1990 and 1991 Conferences. Pay particular attention to an address by Marcel Kinsbourne, M.D., on psychostimulant medication at the 1991 Conference.

You will add to your education by reading the literature you are going to require parents to read. Do not advise or provide anything you have not read. I suggest for parents either *Your Hyperactive Child,* by Barbara Ingersoll, Ph.D., or Edna D. Copeland, Ph.D., and Valerie L. Love's, M.Ed., book, *Attention, Please!* These are fairly good-size books. I want parents to make the effort to get through one or the other, for reading a pamphlet will not provide the understanding necessary to care appropriately for the child with ADD. (Remember—to understand it is to treat it.) After you read these books you will be able to judge which one will be most appropriate for particular parents. I usually have a few copies to loan out, but most often recommend purchase.

> *Attention, Please!: A Comprehensive Guide for Successfully Parenting Children with Attention Disorders and Hyperactivity*, Edna D. Copeland, Ph.D., and Valerie L. Love, M.Ed., SPI Press, P.O. Box 12389, Atlanta, Georgia 30355-2389, (800) 526-5952 (352 pages hard cover).

> *Your Hyperactive Child: A Parent's Guide to Living with Attention Deficit Disorder*, Barbara Ingersoll, Ph.D., A.D.D. Warehouse (Doubleday Book also available in many book stores), 300 Northwest 70th Avenue, Suite 102, Plantation, Florida 33317, (800) 233-9273 (209 pages soft cover).

I will, on occasion, advise or provide videotapes for those who cannot or will not read a book, but generally I prefer that parents become more actively involved by making the effort to absorb written information. Videotapes are excellent for grandparents, other relatives, and close friends. (Obtaining a check or credit-card imprint usually insures return of your materials. If parents decide to keep them, you can order more.)

Once I have made the diagnosis of ADD, I loan my young patient information regarding the disorder that he or she can understand.

My favorite is:

> *Putting on the Brakes.* Patricia O. Quinn, M.D., and Judith Stern, M.A., Pediatric Development Center, 3268 Arcadia Place N.W., Washington, D.C. 20015, (202) 966-1561 (64 pages soft cover).

Others include:

> *Shelly the Hyperactive Turtle.* Deborah Moss, A.D.D. Warehouse #2281 (24 pages soft cover).

> *Otto Learns About His Medicine.* Matthew Galvin, M.D., A.D.D. Warehouse #1870 (28 pages soft cover).

> *Eagle Eyes.* Jeanne Gehret, M.A., A.D.D. Warehouse #2180 (30 pages soft cover).

Jumpin' Johnny Get Back To Work: A Child's Guide to ADHD/Hyperactivity. Michael Gordon, Ph.D., A.D.D. Warehouse #0650 (30 pages soft cover).

Obtain these from:

A.D.D. Warehouse (send for catalog of ADD instructional material), 300 Northwest 70th Avenue, Suite 102, Plantation, FL 33317, (800) 233-9273.

Video: "It's Just Attention Disorder: A Video for Kids." Sam Goldstein, Ph.D., and Michael Goldstein, M.D., MTV format acquaints the child with evaluation and treatment (30 minutes), Neurology Learning and Behavior Center, 230 South 500 East, Suite 100, Salt Lake City, UT 84102, (801) 532-1486.

I frequently furnish my patients' teachers the Goldstein ADD Guide for Teachers to familiarize them with the subject:

A Teacher's Guide: Attention Deficit Hyperactivity Disorder. Sam Goldstein, Ph.D., and Michael Goldstein, M.D. (24 pages soft cover), A.D.D. Warehouse #1567 (package of 10).

In talks I give to teachers I recommend purchase of Copeland and Love's handbook which discusses in detail the classroom management of the child with ADD:

Attention Without Tension: A Teacher's Handbook on Attention Disorders. Edna D. Copeland, Ph.D., and Valerie L. Love, M.Ed. (190 pages spiral bound, soft cover).

There is an excellent companion 3-hour, 2-cassette videotape program entitled "Attention Disorders: The School's Vital Role."

These items can be obtained from:

3 C's of Childhood Inc., P.O. Box 12389, Atlanta, GA 30355-2389 (send for catalog of ADD instructional material), (800) 526-5952.

The computer is rapidly becoming a necessary tool for the appropriate education of the child with ADD. Its use takes advantage of the circumstances that modify the condition and improve the goodness of fit, *i.e.*, one-to-one instruction, a quiet environment, and interesting and immediate feedback. Keep your eye on a company in Charlotte, North Carolina called RMI (Robertson Marketing Inc.). This started out as a Ma-and-Pa computer company, but, because Buzz and Ellen Robertson have two children with ADD, they began to assemble appropriate software and have developed a computer learning technique (triangle of learning).

Write or call them. They will send you information about what they are doing and an excellent software catalog of programs they've found to be effective in educating the child with ADD.

> Robertson Marketing, Inc., Educational Service Division, 803 Pressley Road, Suite 104, Charlotte, NC 28217-1971, (704) 527-5141.

To assist parents in developing an effective behavior management program I advise purchase of Tom Phelan's *1-2-3 Magic* booklet and will often loan them a copy of the videotape.

> *1-2-3- Magic: Training Your Preschooler and Preteen to Do What You Want Them To Do.* Thomas W. Phelan, Ph.D. (57 pages soft cover).

> Video: *1-2-3 Magic.* Thomas W. Phelan, Ph.D. (120 minutes on one cassette).

> Obtain from:

> > Child Management, 800 Roosevelt Road, Building B, Glen Ellyn, IL 60137, (800) 442-4453.

Responsibility and Organization

Teaching responsibility and organization are important, though often neglected, facets of the treatment of the child with attention deficit disorder. I often recommend that parents obtain the Responsibility Programs and the *Organization Notebook for Class and Homework* developed by 3 C's of Childhood, Inc. in Atlanta, GA.

> "Chipper Bear® Responsibility Program Ages 3-7." This comes complete with an audio program, full color chart and the

sought-after Chipper Chips®.

"Responsibility Program Ages 7-12" with a separate teen chart. This contains an audioprogram, responsibility charts and family organization calendar.

These can be obtained from:

3 C's of Childhood, Inc., P.O. Box 12389, Atlanta, GA 30355-2389, (800) 526-5952.

You should have available some rating scales. I most often use the *DuPaul ADHD Rating Scale* (during my initial interview), the *Copeland Symptom Checklist* (following my initial interview), and the *Achenbach Child Behavior Checklist-CBCL* (if I am at all suspicious of a mimic or co-morbidity)

ADHD Rating Scale. George DuPaul, Ph.D., Child Outpatient Psychiatry, 37 Harvard Street, Worcester, MA 01609, (508) 791-5100.

Copeland Symptom Checklist for Attention Deficit Disorders. SPI Press, (800) 526-5952 (See Appendix F).

Achenbach Child Behavior Checklist and Manual. Thomas M. Achenbach, Ph.D., Department of Psychiatry, University of Vermont, 1 South Prospect Street, Burlington, VT 05401, (802) 656-4563.

Also equip your practice with something about Tourette Syndrome. The easiest way to do this is to write the Tourette Syndrome Association and request:

"Questions and Answers on Tourette Syndrome" (small pamphlet for parents).

"Guide to the Diagnosis and Treatment of Tourette Syndrome," "Tourette Syndrome: Recent Advances," (paper-covered booklets for you).

These can be obtained at no charge from the Tourette Syndrome Association, 42-40 Bell Blvd., Bayside, NY 11361, (718) 224-2999.

Some forms will be necessary. Copies of the forms I use are provided in Appendix I:

> *Request for School Records/Reciprocal*
> *Physician Information Form*
> *School Medication Request*
> *Request for Medication Change*
> *Medication Side Effects*

A sturdy rack to hold all of the ADD instructional material and forms you will require in your work is very helpful.

Join CH.A.D.D. (Children with Attention Deficit Disorder). An extremely well-run parent/professional organization supporting the needs of the child with ADD. Membership entitles you to receive a very informative, well-written newsletter. The article, *Medical Management: Commonly Asked Questions*," in Appendix L is from that newsletter.

CH.A.D.D., 499 Northwest 70th Avenue, Suite 308, Plantation, FL 33317, (305) 587-3700.

APPENDIX C

OTHER PUBLICATIONS, VIDEOS AND RESOURCES

For general information

Hyperactivity and Attention Deficit Disorder. Thomas Phelan, Ph.D., Child Management, Glen Ellyn, IL.

Why Johnny Can't Concentrate. Robert A. Moss, M.D., A.D.D. Warehouse #0435.

Video: "Understanding Attention Disorders." Edna D. Copeland, Ph.D., 3 C's of Childhood, Inc. 45 minutes.

Video: "Attention Deficit Hyperactivity Disorder." Thomas Phelan, Ph.D., Child Management, Glen Ellyn, IL.

Medication

Ritalin: Theory and Patient Management. Laurence L. Greenhill, M.D., and Betty B. Osman, Ph.D. (eds.), Mary Ann Liebert Publishers, 1651 3rd Avenue, New York, NY 10128, (212) 289-2300.

Medications for Attention Deficit Disorders (ADHD/ADD) and Related Medical Problems: A Comprehensive Handbook. Edna D. Copeland, Ph.D., SPI Press, P. O. Box 12389, Atlanta, GA 30305-12389, (800) 526-5952.

For Schools

Attention Without Tension: A Teacher's Handbook on Attention Disorders. Edna D. Copeland, Ph.D., and Valerie L. Love, M.Ed., 3 C's of Childhood, Inc.

The ADD Hyperactivity Workbook. Harvey C. Parker, Ph.D., A.D.D. Warehouse #0954.

Video: "Educating Inattentive Children." Sam Goldstein, Ph.D., and Michael Goldstein, M.D., A.D.D. Warehouse #1563, 120 minutes.

From Parents about their ADD children

Maybe You Know My Kid: A Parent's Guide to Identifying, Understanding, and Helping Your Child with Attention Deficit Hyperactivity Disorder. Mary Cahill Fowler, A.D.D. Warehouse #2429.

Sometimes I Get All Scribbly. Maureen Bissen Neuville, Crystal Press, 1624 Mississippi Street, La Crosse, WI 54601, (608) 782-3126.

Behavior

Defiant Children: A Clinician's Manual for Parent Training. Russell A. Barkley, Ph.D., A.D.D. Warehouse #0778A. Set of five parent-teacher assignment books, A.D.D. Warehouse #0778B.

Winning the Homework War. Kathleen Anesko and Frederick Levine, Arco - Simon and Schuster; distributed by Prentice Hall.

Back in Control: How To Get Your Children To Behave. Gregory Bodenhamer, Prentice Hall.

Living With Children: New Methods for Parents and Teachers. Gerald R. Patterson, Ph.D., Research Press.

The Good Kid Book: How To Solve the 16 Most Common Behavior Problems. Howard N. Sloane, A.D.D. Warehouse #1973.

Learning Disabilities

Diagnosis and Management of Learning Disabilities: An Interdisciplinary/Lifespan Approach. Frank R. Brown, III, M.D., Ph.D., Elizabeth Aylward, Ph.D., and Barbara K. Keogh, Ph.D. San Diego, CA: Singular Publishing Group, Inc., 1992.

The Misunderstood Child: A Guide for Parents of Learning-Disabled Children. Larry B. Silver, M.D. New York: McGraw Hill Book Company, 1984 (discusses the combination of ADD with LD).

Keeping A Head In School: A Student's Book About Learning Abilities and Learning Disorders. Mel Levine, M.D., A.D.D. Warehouse #3465. A book written for students with learning problems.

Video: "How Difficult Can This Be?" Richard Lavoie. Graphic depiction of what it is like to be learning disabled.

All parents of children with learning disabilities and every teacher in the country should see this tape.

PBS Video, 1320 Braddock Place, Alexandria, VA 22314, (703) 739-5380 (70 minutes single cassette).

APPENDIX D

INTAKE CHECKLIST

I use this checklist to guide my questioning at the time of the initial visit with parents and child. I do not have parents fill out any type of rating scale or provide answers on a questionnaire before I have a chance to meet with them. I am very interested in how parents reply to questions, how they deal with their youngster and what their affect is. I also wish to develop some dialogue with them regarding their answers to certain questions.

ADD INTAKE CHECKLIST

Stephen C. Copps, M.D.
Comprehensive Child Care Center Gundersen Clinic

Name   School and Grade
Referred by   Address
Age   Sex   Teacher
Primary Medical Care   Other Contact Person
                              Position

	True (Yes)	False (No)	?
Medical History			
Pregnancy problems	[ ]	[ ]	[ ]
Labor/delivery problems	[ ]	[ ]	[ ]
Premature	[ ]	[ ]	[ ]
Small for gestational age	[ ]	[ ]	[ ]
Neonatal complications	[ ]	[ ]	[ ]
Did not leave hospital with mother	[ ]	[ ]	[ ]
Serious illness	[ ]	[ ]	[ ]
Serious accident or injury	[ ]	[ ]	[ ]
Convulsions	[ ]	[ ]	[ ]
Periods of unconsciousness	[ ]	[ ]	[ ]
Hospitalizations	[ ]	[ ]	[ ]
Allergies	[ ]	[ ]	[ ]
Abnormal growth	[ ]	[ ]	[ ]
Delayed motor milestones	[ ]	[ ]	[ ]
Delayed speech milestones	[ ]	[ ]	[ ]
Medications	[ ]	[ ]	[ ]
Infant Temperament			
Colic	[ ]	[ ]	[ ]
Fussy/irritable	[ ]	[ ]	[ ]
Erratic sleeping habits	[ ]	[ ]	[ ]
Difficult to console	[ ]	[ ]	[ ]
Jittery	[ ]	[ ]	[ ]
Feeding problems	[ ]	[ ]	[ ]
Toddler Temperament			
Into everything	[ ]	[ ]	[ ]
Temper tantrums	[ ]	[ ]	[ ]
Difficult to manage	[ ]	[ ]	[ ]
Screamer	[ ]	[ ]	[ ]

	True (Yes)	False (No)	?
Preschool Performance			
Fine-motor difficulty (coloring within the lines)	[ ]	[ ]	[ ]
Gross motor difficulty (clumsy)	[ ]	[ ]	[ ]
Physically aggressive	[ ]	[ ]	[ ]
Bossy	[ ]	[ ]	[ ]
Accident prone	[ ]	[ ]	[ ]
Does not get along with others	[ ]	[ ]	[ ]
A loner	[ ]	[ ]	[ ]
School Performance			
Academic difficulty	[ ]	[ ]	[ ]
Title I help	[ ]	[ ]	[ ]
LD	[ ]	[ ]	[ ]
Other special help	[ ]	[ ]	[ ]
Poor handwriting	[ ]	[ ]	[ ]
Doesn't work to potential	[ ]	[ ]	[ ]
Negative school behavior	[ ]	[ ]	[ ]
Immature	[ ]	[ ]	[ ]
Family History			
Mother - Occupation _____			
‾‾			
Didn't finish high school	[ ]	[ ]	[ ]
Special help	[ ]	[ ]	[ ]
Academic difficulty	[ ]	[ ]	[ ]
Speech or language difficulty	[ ]	[ ]	[ ]
Doesn't read for enjoyment	[ ]	[ ]	[ ]
Poor health	[ ]	[ ]	[ ]
ADD or hyperactive	[ ]	[ ]	[ ]
Father - Occupation _____			
‾‾			
Didn't finish high school	[ ]	[ ]	[ ]
Special help	[ ]	[ ]	[ ]
Academic difficulty	[ ]	[ ]	[ ]
Speech or language difficulty	[ ]	[ ]	[ ]
Doesn't read for enjoyment	[ ]	[ ]	[ ]
Poor health	[ ]	[ ]	[ ]
ADD or hyperactive	[ ]	[ ]	[ ]
Siblings			
Academic difficulty	[ ]	[ ]	[ ]
Behavior difficulty	[ ]	[ ]	[ ]
Poor health	[ ]	[ ]	[ ]

	True (Yes)	False (No)	?
ADD or hyperactive	[ ]	[ ]	[ ]
Unmarried mother	[ ]	[ ]	[ ]
Divorce	[ ]	[ ]	[ ]
Mother remarried	[ ]	[ ]	[ ]
Father remarried	[ ]	[ ]	[ ]
Absent parent	[ ]	[ ]	[ ]
Parent deceased	[ ]	[ ]	[ ]
Alcoholism	[ ]	[ ]	[ ]
Drug addiction	[ ]	[ ]	[ ]
Mental illness	[ ]	[ ]	[ ]
Sociopathic behavior (arrests, jail, etc.)	[ ]	[ ]	[ ]
Child abuse	[ ]	[ ]	[ ]
Sexual abuse	[ ]	[ ]	[ ]

Psychological Concerns

Hears things that aren't there	[ ]	[ ]	[ ]
Sees things that aren't there	[ ]	[ ]	[ ]
Seems depressed	[ ]	[ ]	[ ]
Seems anxious	[ ]	[ ]	[ ]
Attempted suicide	[ ]	[ ]	[ ]
Seen by psychologist	[ ]	[ ]	[ ]
Seen by psychiatrist	[ ]	[ ]	[ ]
Extremely moody	[ ]	[ ]	[ ]
Sleep disturbance	[ ]	[ ]	[ ]
A real loner	[ ]	[ ]	[ ]
Marked fantasy	[ ]	[ ]	[ ]
Severe aggression	[ ]	[ ]	[ ]
Parental rejection	[ ]	[ ]	[ ]
Persistent worrier	[ ]	[ ]	[ ]
Urge to constantly repeat activities or thoughts	[ ]	[ ]	[ ]
Pressured speech	[ ]	[ ]	[ ]
Prolonged tantrums	[ ]	[ ]	[ ]

ADD Characteristics: (DSM-III-R):
(You may substitute the DuPaul ADHD Rating Scale for this section)

	True (Yes)	False (No)	?
Often fidgets	[ ]	[ ]	[ ]
Difficulty remaining seated	[ ]	[ ]	[ ]
Easily distracted	[ ]	[ ]	[ ]
Difficulty awaiting turn	[ ]	[ ]	[ ]
Difficulty following through on instructions	[ ]	[ ]	[ ]
Often blurts out answers	[ ]	[ ]	[ ]
Difficulty sustaining attention	[ ]	[ ]	[ ]
Difficulty playing quietly	[ ]	[ ]	[ ]
Talks excessively	[ ]	[ ]	[ ]
Shifts from one uncompleted task to another	[ ]	[ ]	[ ]
Often interrupts	[ ]	[ ]	[ ]
Often loses things	[ ]	[ ]	[ ]
Does not seem to listen	[ ]	[ ]	[ ]
Engages in physically dangerous activity	[ ]	[ ]	[ ]

Other ADD Characteristics

	True (Yes)	False (No)	?
Remarkable memory for remote events	[ ]	[ ]	[ ]
Extraordinary attention to detail	[ ]	[ ]	[ ]
Takes it all in at one time	[ ]	[ ]	[ ]
Marked fluctuation in performance	[ ]	[ ]	[ ]
Flight of ideas	[ ]	[ ]	[ ]
Overreacts	[ ]	[ ]	[ ]
Requires instant gratification	[ ]	[ ]	[ ]
Marked intensity	[ ]	[ ]	[ ]
Little respect for boundaries	[ ]	[ ]	[ ]
Poor organizational skills	[ ]	[ ]	[ ]
Failure to anticipate consequences	[ ]	[ ]	[ ]
Difficulty with transitions	[ ]	[ ]	[ ]
Complains of boredom	[ ]	[ ]	[ ]
Brutally frank	[ ]	[ ]	[ ]
Restless sleeper	[ ]	[ ]	[ ]
Night terrors	[ ]	[ ]	[ ]

	True (Yes)	False (No)	?
Oppositional Defiant Characteristics: (DSM-III-R)*			
Often loses temper	[ ]	[ ]	[ ]
Argues with adults	[ ]	[ ]	[ ]
Defies adult rules	[ ]	[ ]	[ ]
Refuses adult requests	[ ]	[ ]	[ ]
Does things to deliberately annoy	[ ]	[ ]	[ ]
Blames others for his/her mistakes	[ ]	[ ]	[ ]
Angry and resentful	[ ]	[ ]	[ ]
Spiteful or vindictive	[ ]	[ ]	[ ]
Uses obscene language	[ ]	[ ]	[ ]

*If more than 5 "yes" answers in this section, ask questions relative to conduct disorder (see Appendix E).

	True (Yes)	False (No)	?
Desirable Traits			
Enthusiastic	[ ]	[ ]	[ ]
Energetic	[ ]	[ ]	[ ]
Artistic	[ ]	[ ]	[ ]
Musical	[ ]	[ ]	[ ]
Athletic	[ ]	[ ]	[ ]
Sensitive to others needs	[ ]	[ ]	[ ]
Inquisitive	[ ]	[ ]	[ ]
Intuitive	[ ]	[ ]	[ ]
Resilient	[ ]	[ ]	[ ]
Attentive to detail	[ ]	[ ]	[ ]
Marvelous imagination	[ ]	[ ]	[ ]
Outgoing	[ ]	[ ]	[ ]
Likable	[ ]	[ ]	[ ]
Good sense of humor	[ ]	[ ]	[ ]
Good talker	[ ]	[ ]	[ ]
Doesn't hold a grudge	[ ]	[ ]	[ ]

NOTES: To consider the diagnosis of ADD, make certain the criteria of the DSM-III-R have been met. I'd use my modifications listed on page 33. To make the diagnosis, I like to see at least 10 *yes* answers under other ADD characteristics and a definite *yes* for remarkable memory for remote events, marked fluctuation in performance and *taking it all in.*

If there are six or more *yes* answers under oppositional defiant characteristics, or a conduct disorder appears to be present, I will consider immediate referral to a child psychologist.

If there is obvious depression, clinical anxiety, suicidal tendencies, possible bipolar disorder, obsessive-compulsive disorder, or hallucinations, I will refer to a child psychiatrist.

Following the initial interview, permission is obtained to get school records. I have both parents independently fill out a Copeland Symptom Checklist and send it back to me.

If there is a family history of emotional problems, alcoholism, drug addiction, sociopathic behavior or there is a *yes* answer to any questions under psychological concerns, I will have both parents fill out an Achenbach Child Behavior Checklist (CBCL).

I find that after I have completed the initial interview, reviewed the completed symptom checklists and read the school records I can accurately make a diagnosis of ADD in approximately 70% of those children who have the condition. This spares, for many, an expensive, in-depth psychological or psychoeducational workup.

APPENDIX E

BEHAVIORS

- DuPaul Rating Scale for ADHD*

- Comparison of ADHD/ODD Behaviors (DSM-III-R)

- Comparison of ADHD/ODD/CD Behaviors (DSM-III-R)

*ADHD and ADD are used interchangeably.

The DuPaul ADHD Rating Scale

Child's Name: _____   Age_____   Grade_____
Completed by: _____
Circle the Number in the Column That Best Describes the Child

	Not at all	Just a Little	Pretty Much	Very Much
1. Often fidgets or squirms in seat	0	1	2	3
2. Has difficulty remaining seated	0	1	2	3
3. Is easily distracted	0	1	2	3
4. Has difficulty awaiting turn in groups	0	1	2	3
5. Often blurts out answers to questions	0	1	2	3
6. Has difficulty following instructions	0	1	2	3
7. Has difficulty sustaining attention to tasks	0	1	2	3
8. Often shifts from one uncompleted activity to another	0	1	2	3
9. Has difficulty playing quietly	0	1	2	3
10. Often talks excessively	0	1	2	3
11. Often interrupts or intrudes on others	0	1	2	3
12. Often does not seem to listen	0	1	2	3
13. Often loses things necessary for tasks	0	1	2	3
14. Often engages in physically dangerous activities without considering consequences	0	1	2	3

Scores of 2 or higher are considered inappropriate for a child's developmental level. The number of items with scores of 2 or above determines whether the child meets the criteria for diagnosis (see page 33). Used by permission of the author.

BEHAVIORAL CHARACTERISTICS DSM-III-R

ADHD Characteristics
(Skill-Deficit Behaviors)

1. Fidgety
2. Difficulty remaining seated
3. Easily distracted
4. Difficulty awaiting turn
5. Difficulty following through on instructions
6. Blurts out answers
7. Difficulty sustaining attention
8. Difficulty playing quietly
9. Talks excessively
10. Shifts from one uncompleted task to another
11. Interrupts
12. Loses things
13. Does not seem to listen
14. Engages in physically dangerous activities

Total = ___

Significant: (See page 33)

Oppositional/Defiant Behaviors
(Noncompliant Behaviors)

1. Loses temper
2. Argues with adults
3. Defies adult rules
4. Refuses adult requests
5. Does things deliberately to annoy
6. Blames others for his/her mistakes
7. Angry and resentful
8. Spiteful or vindictive
9. Swears or uses obscene language

Total = ___

Significant: Disturbance of at least 6 months, during which at least five are present.

Diagnostic and Statistical Manual of Mental Disorders: Third Edition, Revised (DSM-III-R). Copyright 1987 by the American Psychiatric Association. Reprinted with publisher's permission.

BEHAVIORAL CHARACTERISTICS FROM THE DSM-III-R

ADHD Characteristics (Incompetent, skill-deficit behaviors) - **No Punishment**	Oppositional/Defiant Behaviors (ODD) (Noncompliant behaviors)	Conduct Disorder Behaviors (CD)
Fidgety ☐	Loses temper ☐	Stealing ☐
Difficulty remaining seated ☐	Argues with adults ☐	Running away from home ☐
Easily distracted ☐	Defies adult rules ☐	Repetitive lying ☐
Difficulty awaiting turn ☐	Refuses adult requests ☐	Fire setting ☐
Difficulty following instructions ☐	Does things to deliberately annoy ☐	Truant from school ☐
Blurts out answers ☐	Blames others for mistakes ☐	Breaking and entering ☐
Difficulty sustaining attention ☐	Resentful ☐	Destroying property ☐
Difficulty playing quietly ☐	Undue anger ☐	Physically cruel to animals ☐
Talks excessively ☐	Spiteful or vindictive ☐	Forced sexual activity ☐
Shifts from one uncompleted task to another ☐	Swears or uses obscene language ☐	Use of weapons in fights ☐
Interrupts ☐		Frequently initiates fights ☐
Loses things ☐		Armed robbery/mugging ☐
Does not seem to listen ☐		Physically cruel to people ☐
Engages in physically dangerous activities ☐		
Total = ___	Total = ___	Total = ___
Significant: (See Page 33)	Significant: Disturbance of at least 6 months, during which at least five are present.	Significant: Disturbance of at least 6 months, during which three are present.

Diagnostic and Statistical Manual of Mental Disorders; Third Edition, Revised (DSM-III-R).
Copyright 1987 by the American Psychiatric Association. Reprinted with publisher's permission.

APPENDIX F

Copeland Symptom Checklist for Attention Deficit Disorders (ADHD and ADD)

Copeland Symptom Checklist for Adult Attention Deficit Disorders (ADHD and ADD)

Scoring for Copeland Checklists

SPI

COPELAND SYMPTOM CHECKLIST FOR ATTENTION DEFICIT DISORDERS

Attention Deficit Hyperactivity Disorder (ADHD)
and Undifferentiated Attention Deficit Disorder (ADD)

This checklist was developed from the experience of many specialists in the field of Attention Deficit Disorders and Hyperactivity. It is designed to help you assess whether your child/student has ADHD or ADD, to what degree, and if so, in which area(s) difficulties are experienced. Please mark all statements. Thank you for your assistance in completing this information.

Name of Child _____ Date _____

Completed by _____

Directions: Place a checkmark (✔) by each item below, indicating the degree to which the behavior is characteristic of your child/student.

* denotes ADD with Hyperactivity (ADHD).
• denotes ADD without Hyperactivity (Undifferentiated ADD)

	Not at all	Just a little	Pretty much	Very much	Score	%
I. INATTENTION/DISTRACTIBILITY						
*• 1. A short attention span, especially for low-interest activities.						
*• 2. Difficulty completing tasks.						
• 3. Daydreaming.						
*• 4. Easily distracted.						
• 5. Nicknames such as: "spacey," or "dreamer."						
*• 6. Engages in much activity but accomplishes little.						
*• 7. Enthusiastic beginnings but poor endings.					= 21	%
II. IMPULSIVITY						
* 1. Excitability.						
*• 2. Low frustration tolerance.						
*• 3. Acts before thinking.						
*• 4. Disorganization.						
*• 5. Poor planning ability.						
*• 6. Excessively shifts from one activity to another.						
* 7. Difficulty in group situations which require patience and taking turns.						
*• 8. Requires much supervision.						
*• 9. Constantly in trouble for deeds of omission as well as deeds of commission.						
*• 10. Frequently interrupts conversations; talks out of turn.					= 30	%
III. ACTIVITY LEVEL PROBLEMS						
A. Overactivity/Hyperactivity						
*• 1. Restlessness — either fidgetiness or being constantly on the go.						
* 2. Diminished need for sleep.						
* 3. Excessive talking.						
* 4. Excessive running, jumping and climbing.						
* 5. Motor restlessness during sleep. Kicks covers off — moves around constantly.						
* 6. Difficulty staying seated at meals, in class, etc. Often walks around classroom.					= 18	%
B. Underactivity						
• 1. Lethargy.						
• 2. Daydreaming, spaciness.						
• 3. Failure to complete tasks.						
*• 4. Inattention.						
*• 5. Poor leadership ability.						
*• 6. Difficulty in learning and performing.					= 18	%
IV. NON-COMPLIANCE						
*• 1. Frequently disobeys.						
*• 2. Argumentative.						
* 3. Disregards socially-accepted standards of behavior.						
• 4. "Forgets" unintentionally.						
5. Uses "forgetting" as an excuse (intentional).					= 15	%

Copyright ©1987 by Edna D. Copeland, Ph.D.

Published by **SPI** Southeastern Psychological Institute, P.O. Box 12389, Atlanta, Georgia 30355-2389

Used by permission of the author.

COPELAND SYMPTOM CHECKLIST FOR ATTENTION DEFICIT DISORDERS (Continued)

	Not at all	Just a little	Pretty much	Very much
V. ATTENTION-GETTING BEHAVIOR				
* 1. Frequently needs to be the center of attention.				
* 2. Constantly asks questions or interrupts.				
* 3. Irritates and annoys siblings, peers and adults.				
* 4. Behaves as the "class clown."				
* 5. Uses bad or rude language to attract attention.				
* 6. Engages in other negative behaviors to attract attention.				
VI. IMMATURITY				
*• 1. Behavior resembles that of a younger child. Responses are typical of children 6 months to 2-plus years younger.				
*• 2. Physical development is delayed.				
*• 3. Prefers younger children and relates better to them.				
*• 4. Emotional reactions are often immature.				
VII. POOR ACHIEVEMENT/COGNITIVE & VISUAL-MOTOR PROBLEMS				
*• 1. Underachieves relative to ability.				
*• 2. Loses books, assignments, etc.				
*• 3. Auditory memory and auditory processing problems.				
*• 4. Learning disabilities/learning problems.				
*• 5. Incomplete assignments.				
*• 6. Academic work completed too quickly.				
*• 7. Academic work completed too slowly.				
*• 8. "Messy" or "sloppy" written work; poor handwriting.				
*• 9. Poor memory for directions, instructions and rote learning.				
VIII. EMOTIONAL DIFFICULTIES				
*• 1. Frequent and unpredictable mood swings.				
*• 2. High levels of irritability.				
* 3. Underreactive to pain/insensitive to danger.				
* 4. Easily overstimulated. Hard to calm down once over-excited.				
*• 5. Low frustration tolerance.				
* 6. Temper tantrums, angry outbursts.				
• 7. Moodiness.				
*• 8. Low self-esteem.				
IX. POOR PEER RELATIONS				
* 1. Hits, bites, or kicks other children.				
* 2. Difficulty following the rules of games and social interactions.				
*• 3. Rejected or avoided by peers.				
• 4. Avoids group activities; a loner.				
* 5. Teases peers and siblings excessively.				
* 6. Bullies or bosses other children.				
X. FAMILY INTERACTION PROBLEMS				
1. Frequent family conflict.				
2. Activities and social gatherings are unpleasant.				
3. Parents argue over discipline since nothing works.				
4. Mother spends hours and hours on homework with ADD child leaving little time for others in family.				
5. Meals are frequently unpleasant.				
6. Arguments occur between parents and child over responsibilities and chores.				
7. Stress is continuous from child's social and academic problems.				
8. Parents, especially mother, feel: ☐ frustrated ☐ hopeless ☐ alone ☐ angry ☐ guilty ☐ afraid for child ☐ helpless ☐ disappointed ☐ sad and depressed				

18 = %
12 = %
27 = %
24 = %
18 = %
24 = %

TOTAL = %
225

Copyright © 1987 by Edna D. Copeland, Ph.D.

7/90 Published by **SPI** Southeastern Psychological Institute. P.O. Box 12389, Atlanta, Georgia 30355-2389

Used by permission of the author.

SPI

COPELAND SYMPTOM CHECKLIST
FOR ADULT ATTENTION DEFICIT DISORDERS

Attention Deficit Hyperactivity Disorder (ADHD)
and Undifferentiated Attention Deficit Disorder (ADD)

This checklist was developed from the experience of many specialists in the field of Attention Disorders and Hyperactivity. It is designed to help determine whether you, or someone you are rating, has ADHD or ADD, to what degree, and if so, in which area(s) difficulties are experienced. Please mark all statements. Thank you for your assistance in completing this information.

Name _____ Date _____

Completed by _____

Directions: Place a checkmark (✓) by each item below, indicating the degree to which the behavior is characteristic of yourself or the adult you are rating.

	Not at all	Just a little	Pretty much	Very much	Score	%
I. INATTENTION/DISTRACTIBILITY, especially						
1. A short attention span, especially for low-interest activities.						
2. Difficulty completing tasks.						
3. Daydreaming.						
4. Easily distracted.						
5. Nicknames such as: "spacey," or "dreamer."						
6. Engages in much activity but accomplishes little.						
7. Enthusiastic beginnings but poor endings.						
					= ___ % 21	
II. IMPULSIVITY						
1. Excitability.						
2. Low frustration tolerance.						
3. Acts before thinking.						
4. Disorganization.						
5. Poor planning ability.						
6. Excessively shifts from one activity to another.						
7. Difficulty in group situations which require patience and taking turns.						
8. Interrupts frequently.						
					= ___ % 24	
III. ACTIVITY LEVEL PROBLEMS						
A. Overactivity/Hyperactivity						
1. Restlessness — either fidgetiness or being constantly on the go.						
2. Diminished need for sleep.						
3. Excessive talking.						
4. Difficulty listening.						
5. Motor restlessness during sleep. Kicks covers off — moves around constantly.						
6. Dislike of situations which require attention & being still—church, lectures, etc.					= ___ % 18	
B. Underactivity						
1. Lethargic.						
2. Daydreaming, spaciness.						
3. Failure to complete tasks.						
4. Inattention.						
5. Lacking in leadership.						
6. Difficulty in getting things done.					= ___ % 18	

Published by SPI Southeastern Psychological Institute, P.O. Box 12389, Atlanta, Georgia 30355-2389

Used by permission of the author.

COPELAND SYMPTOM CHECKLIST FOR ADULT ATTENTION DEFICIT DISORDERS (Continued)

	Not at all	Just a little	Pretty much	Very much
IV. NONCOMPLIANCE				
1. Does not cooperate. Determined to do things own way.				
2. Argumentative.				
3. Disregards socially-accepted behavioral expectations.				
4. "Forgets" unintentionally.				
5. "Forgets" as an excuse (intentionally).				

         ____ = ____%
        15

	Not at all	Just a little	Pretty much	Very much
V. UNDERACHIEVEMENT/DISORGANIZATION/LEARNING PROBLEMS				
1. Underachievement in relation to ability.				
2. Frequent job changes.				
3. Loses things — keys, wallet, lists, belongings, etc.				
4. Auditory memory and auditory processing problems.				
5. Learning disabilities or learning problems.				
6. Poor handwriting.				
7. "Messy" or "sloppy" work.				
8. Work assignments are often not completed satisfactorily.				
9. Rushes through work.				
10. Works too slowly.				
11. Procrastinates. Bills, taxes, etc., put off until the last minute.				

         ____ = ____%
        33

	Not at all	Just a little	Pretty much	Very much
VI. EMOTIONAL DIFFICULTIES				
1. Frequent and unpredictable mood swings.				
2. Irritability.				
3. Underreactive to pain/insensitive to danger.				
4. Easily overstimulated. Hard to stop once "revved up."				
5. Low frustration tolerance. Excessive emotional reaction to frustrating situations.				
6. Angry outbursts.				
7. Moodiness/lack of energy.				
8. Low self-esteem.				
9. Immaturity.				

         ____ = ____%
        27

	Not at all	Just a little	Pretty much	Very much
VII. POOR PEER RELATIONS				
1. Difficulty following the rules of social interactions.				
2. Rejected or avoided by peers.				
3. Avoids group activities; a loner.				
4. "Bosses" other people. Wants to be the leader.				
5. Critical of others.				

         ____ = ____%
        15

	Not at all	Just a little	Pretty much	Very much
VIII. IMPAIRED FAMILY RELATIONSHIPS				
1. Easily frustrated with spouse or children. Overreacts. May punish children too severely.				
2. Sees things from own point of view. Does not negotiate differences well.				
3. Underdeveloped sense of responsibility.				
4. Poor manager of money.				
5. Unreasonable; demanding.				
6. Spends excessive amount of time at work because of inefficiency, leaving little time for family.				

         ____ = ____%
        18

        TOTAL ____ = ____%
        189

7/90   Published by **SPI** Southeastern Psychological Institute, P.O. Box 12389, Atlanta, Georgia 30355-2389

Used by permission of the author.

S**PI**

SCORING THE COPELAND SYMPTOM CHECKLIST
FOR ATTENTION DEFICIT DISORDERS (ADHD/ADD)

(Child/Adolescent Checklist and Adult Checklist)

1. Scores for each category are as follows:

   Not at all = 0;   Just a little = 1;   Pretty much = 2;   Very much = 3

2. Each check receives a score from 0 - 3. Add the checks in each category. That score is placed over the total possible.
   Example:

	0 Not at all	1 Just a little	2 Pretty much	3 Very much	Score	%
* denotes ADD with Hyperactivity (ADHD). • denotes ADD without Hyperactivity (Undifferentiated ADD)						
I. INATTENTION/DISTRACTIBILITY						
* • 1. A short attention span, especially for low-interest activities.				✔		
* • 2. Difficulty completing tasks.			✔			
• 3. Daydreaming.		✔				
* • 4. Easily distracted.				✔		
• 5. Nicknames such as: "spacey," or "dreamer."		✔				
* • 6. Engages in much activity but accomplishes little.				✔		
* • 7. Enthusiastic beginnings but poor endings.				✔	16 = 76 % / 21	
II. IMPULSIVITY						
* 1. Excitability.				✔		
* • 2. Low frustration tolerance.				✔		
* • 3. Acts before thinking.				✔		
* • 4. Disorganization.			✔			
* • 5. Poor planning ability.			✔			
* • 6. Excessively shifts from one activity to another.				✔		
* 7. Difficulty in group situations which require patience and taking turns.				✔		
* • 8. Requires much supervision.				✔		
* • 9. Constantly in trouble for deeds of omission as well as deeds of commission.			✔			
* • 10. Frequently interrupts conversations; talks out of turn.				✔	27 = 90 % / 30	

3. Compute the percentage for each category.

   Significance:*

   Scores between 35-49% suggest mild to moderate difficulties.

   Scores between 50-69% suggest moderate to severe difficulties.

   Scores above 70% suggest major interference.

   (*These scores represent clinical significance. The scale is currently being normed and statistical data should be available soon.)

   Children, adolescents and adults may have difficulties in only one area or in all ten. Those with undifferentiated ADD on the more daydreaming, inattentive, anxious end of the ADD continuum frequently manifest difficulties only in the "Inattention/Distractibility", "Underactivity", and the "Underachievement" categories, while those with overactive, impulsive ADHD will have difficulties in many more areas of their lives.

Used by permission of the author.

APPENDIX G

ATTENTION DEFICIT DISORDER

A Common Profile Age 0-5

One or both parents had some difficulty in school. One, often the father, does not read for enjoyment, and demonstrates impulsive behavior.

There is no family history of significant mental or emotional illness. No nervous breakdowns.

There were no pregnancy, labor or delivery complications; neonatal course was unremarkable. Gross-motor developmental milestones were well within normal limits, but the infant was described as being colicky and fussy with feeding difficulties and erratic sleeping habits.

The mother became increasingly frustrated, for she was unable to satisfy the needs of her own child and, as a consequence, felt increasingly guilty.

As the child approached two, mother's guilt precluded effective child management. She was unable to be effective with the child and began to harbor resentment. She then felt guilty about the resentment and let the child get away with socially inappropriate behavior. Maddening physical activity increased; the child was in constant motion; and the mother was told that all two-year-old boys act that way. *The Guilt increased.*

At three the child was placed in a nursery school, which gave mother a little badly needed respite but there the child had to be the boss, never sat still and couldn't get along with his peers. The child was described as *accident prone.*

At four the problems persisted and it was noted that he had difficulty cutting out simple shapes and coloring between the lines (deficit in fine-motor performance).

In kindergarten he wouldn't sit on the mat, interrupted constantly, was physically aggressive and had some difficulty with pre-reading skills. The teacher may have become suspicious of the possibility of a developmental problem.

In first grade he is described as being immature and may be having difficulty learning to read. He is hyperactive and does not conform to the classroom rules for behavior.

The child exhibits marked lability of behavior at home as well as school. He operates best in a quiet environment on a one-to-one basis. He often demonstrates a good attention span for those things that hold his interest such as Saturday morning cartoons on TV but has very poor selective attention to task.

He tremendously over-reacts to external stimulation—visual as well as auditory. He's stimulus bound.

Tests may reveal deficiencies in visual-motor perception. He has an excellent memory for remote events, but often can't remember what he has just been told. He has some difficulty with rapid alternating movements and sequential finger tapping. Deep and superficial reflexes are normal. There are no pathologic reflexes. Though motor developmental milestones have been within normal limits, he is somewhat clumsy. Early math skills may be good and he may demonstrate an interest in music, especially rhythm. He often attends to the most minute detail in his drawing. He often becomes very absorbed in minute details and misses the big picture.

Though physically overactive and aggressive, he rarely is mean. He shows remorse when reprimanded, though often is described as a *bad kid*. Social skills are inadequate. He experiences failure after failure academically as well as socially. No one understands him. Everyone tells him he is smart and can do it if he would only try. He can't measure up. His self-image, as well as that of his parents, deteriorates and more and more secondary emotional problems become manifest. As the child gets older, it is much more difficult to determine which came first, the attention deficit disorder or the emotional problems.

He becomes the victim of a system that doesn't understand the biologic nature of the disability and continues to heap guilt upon the parents for having such a misbehaved youngster.

APPENDIX H

TREATMENT OF ADD

1. Educate (To understand it is to treat it)

    A. Parents
    B. Teachers
    C. Child

2. Medicate

3. Manage Behavior

4. Teach Responsibility

5. Encourage Self-Image Enhancement

6. Provide Environmental Modifications

7. Instruct in Social Competency

8. Insure Effective School Program

    A. Behavior
    B. Learning Deficits

9. Attend to Co-Morbidities

10. Attend to Family Problems

11. Attend Support Group Meetings

APPENDIX I

ATTENTION DEFICIT DISORDER FORMS

1. *Request for School Records/Reciprocal Physician Information Form*

2. *School Medication Request*

3. *Request for Medication Change*

4. *Medication Side Effects*

REQUEST FOR SCHOOL RECORDS*

Name   School and Grade

Teacher   Address

Position   Other Contact Person

I am caring for _____, a student of yours. I would appreciate receiving from you copies of the following school records beginning _____ to the present time.

Student Support Services Report	[ ]
IEP	[ ]
Psychological/Psychoeducational Evaluation	[ ]
OT Evaluation including perceptual testing	[ ]
Gross-Motor Performance	[ ]
Vision Screen	[ ]
Hearing Screen	[ ]
Report Cards	[ ]
Teacher Observations	[ ]
Grade Level	
Math	[ ]
Reading	[ ]
Spelling	[ ]

Physician's Signature   Printed Name

Address   Phone Number

I grant permission for the school to release the records requested. I grant permission for the physician named to share information from my child's medical record with the school.

_____   _____

Signature of parent or guardian   Date

*This is a reciprocal form used also for the physician to share medical information with the school.

ATTENTION DEFICIT DISORDER
SCHOOL MEDICATION REQUEST

Name of Student   Age

School   Grade

I am caring for this student who has an attention deficit. I request that you administer the following medication in school at the times specified.

Name of Medication_____

Dose_____   No. of tablets or capsules_____   Time_____
Dose_____   No. of tablets or capsules_____   Time_____
Dose_____   No. of tablets or capsules_____   Time_____

Anticipated benefits include increased sustained attention, decreased impulsivity and decreased distractibility. This medication is not a tranquilizer or mood-altering agent, and it cannot be expected to significantly alter oppositional defiant behavior.

Please notify me at once should you notice any abnormalities of large muscle movement or posturing (dystonia), or note any evidence of personality change.

It is expected that this medication, when the proper dose is obtained, will significantly enhance your student's performance. The improvement should be readily detectable.

Thank you for your cooperation. I will notify you of any medication change and will inform you when I wish the medication to be discontinued.

Signature   Phone Number

Physician's Printed Name   Date

ATTENTION DEFICIT DISORDER
REQUEST FOR MEDICATION CHANGE

Name of Student: Age:

School:
Grade:

This student is presently taking the medication_____
at school at time(s) indicated_____

Please make the following change(s):

	Yes	No
Medication change	( )	( )
Dose change	( )	( )
Time change	( )	( )

Medication:_____

Dose_____ No. of tablets or capsules_____ Time_____
Dose_____ No. of tablets or capsules_____ Time_____
Dose_____ No. of tablets or capsules_____ Time_____

Signature

Physician Printed Name

Phone Number

Date

ATTENTION DEFICIT DISORDER
MEDICATION SIDE EFFECTS

Name   Physician

Medication   Dosage and Time(s)

	None	Some	Quite a bit	Very Much
Appetite decrease	—	—	—	—
Sleeping difficulty	—	—	—	—
Nightmares	—	—	—	—
Whiny	—	—	—	—
Crying	—	—	—	—
Abdominal pain	—	—	—	—
Headaches	—	—	—	—
Sadness	—	—	—	—
Feeling of unreality (don't ask)	—	—	—	—
Hair loss	—	—	—	—
Eye blinking	—	—	—	—
Facial grimacing	—	—	—	—
Small-muscle, abnormal movements Sporadic involuntary tics	—	—	—	—
**Large-muscle, abnormal movements or posturing (Dystonia)	—	—	—	—
**Personality change Student has become	—	—	—	—
*Lethargic	—	—	—	—
*Withdrawn	—	—	—	—
*Sullen	—	—	—	—
*Irritable	—	—	—	—

*Probably indicates too much medication.

**Notify Physician At Once.

APPENDIX J

It is hoped that ADD will serve as a catalyst to break down the barriers that exist between education and medicine, between the physician and the psychologist, between the psychologist and the psychiatrist. It is imperative that we always do what is in the best interest of the child, not what is in the imagined best interest of a self-serving profession, facility or bureaucracy.

GUIDELINES FOR INTERDISCIPLINARY COOPERATION

1. I will learn your language and I will teach you mine.

2. I will ask for your perceptions and feedback to learn more of what you know and to challenge my own timeworn position.

3. I will share my professional strengths and my weaknesses with you so that we both can grow.

4. I will not withhold "disciplinary secrets" from you or cling tenaciously to my turf; but I will tell you when I am feeling that you are stepping on my toes and I want you to do the same for me.

5. I will confront you, challenge you, listen to you and learn from you. I will expect you to do the same for me.

We have used this as a code of conduct in our Comprehensive Child Care Center for years. I cannot remember its origin, but I believe it appeared in either a physical or occupational therapy journal. If you wrote this, please write to me, for I would love to give you the credit you deserve, but most of all I would like to talk to you and learn from you.

APPENDIX K

UNITED STATES DEPARTMENT OF EDUCATION
Office of Special Education and Rehabilitation Services

The Assistant Secretary

MEMORANDUM

Date: September 16, 1991

To: Chief State School Officers

From: Robert R. Davila
          Assistant Secretary
          Office of Special Education
            and Rehabilitation Services

          Michael L. Williams
          Assistant Secretary
          Office of Civil Rights

          John T. MacDonald
          Assistant Secretary
          Office of Elementary
            and Secondary Education

Subject: Clarification of Policy to Address the Needs of
          Children with Attention Deficit Disorders within
          General and/or Special Education

EXCERPTS

PL 94-142 (Individuals with Disabilities Education Act)
II-B   Eligibility for Part B services under the
        "Other Health Impaired" Category

The list of chronic or acute health problems included within the
definition of "other health impaired" in the Part B regulations is
not exhaustive. The term "other health impaired" includes chronic
or acute impairments that result in limited alertness, which
adversely affects educational performance. Thus, children with

ADD should be classified as eligible for services under the "other health impaired" category in instances where the ADD is a chronic or acute health problem that results in limited alertness, which adversely   affects educational performance.   In other words, children with ADD, where the ADD is a chronic or acute health problem resulting in limited alertness, may be considered disabled under Part B solely on the basis of this disorder within the "other health impaired" category in situations where special education and related services are needed because of the ADD.

IV-B Programs and Services Under Section 504 (Rehabilitation
     Act)
     Paragraphs 3-6

Should it be determined that the child with ADD is handicapped for purposes of Section 504 and needs only adjustments in the regular classroom, rather than special education, those adjustments are required by Section 504.   A range of strategies is available to meet the educational needs of children with ADD.

Regular classroom teachers are important in identifying the appropriate educational adaptations and interventions for many children with ADD.

SEAs and LEAs should take the necessary steps to promote coordination between special and regular education problems. Steps also should be taken to train regular education teachers and other personnel to develop their awareness about ADD and its manifestations and the adaptations that can be implemented in regular education programs to address the instructional needs of those children.   Examples of adaptations in regular education programs could include the following:

> Providing   a   structured   learning   environment;
> repeating and simplifying instructions about in-class
> and homework assignments; supplementing verbal
> instructions with visual instructions; using behavioral
> management techniques; adjusting class schedules;
> modifying   test   delivery;   using   tape   recorders,
> computer-aided instruction, and other audio-visual
> equipment; selecting modified textbooks; and tailoring
> homework assignments.

Medical Management of Children with Attention Deficit Disorders
Commonly Asked Questions

by

Children with Attention Deficit Disorders (CH.A.D.D.)
American Academy of Child and Adolescent Psychiatry (AACAP)

Harvey C. Parker, Ph.D.
CH.A.D.D., Executive Director

George Storm, M.D.
CH.A.D.D., Professional Advisory Board

Committee of Community Psychiatry and Consultation to Agencies of AACAP
Theodore A. Petti, M.D., M.P.H., Chairperson
Virginia Q. Anthony, AACAP, Executive Director

This article may be reproduced and distributed without written permission. Tear out for easy use.

1. What is an Attention Deficit Disorder.

Attention deficit disorder (ADD), also known as attention deficit hyperactivity disorder (ADHD), is a treatable disorder which affects approximately three to five per cent of the population. Inattentiveness, impulsivity, and oftentimes, hyperactivity, are common characteristics of the disorder. Boys with ADD tend to outnumber girls by three to one, although ADD in girls is underidentified.

Some common symptoms of ADD are:
1. Excessively fidgets or squirms
2. Difficulty remaining seated
3. Easily distracted
4. Difficulty awaiting turn in games
5. Blurts out answers to questions
6. Difficulty following instructions
7. Difficulty sustaining attention

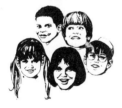

8. Shifts from one activity to another
9. Difficulty playing quietly
10. Often talks excessively
11. Often interrupts
12. Often doesn't listen to what is said
13. Often loses things
14. Often engages in dangerous activities

However, you don't have to be hyperactive to have an attention deficit disorder. In fact, up to 30% of children with ADD are not hyperactive at all, but still have a lot of trouble focusing attention.

2. How can we tell if a child has ADD?

Many factors can cause children to have problems paying attention besides an attention deficit disorder. Family problems, stress, discouragement, drugs, physical illness, and learning difficulties can all cause problems that look like ADD, but really aren't. To accurately identify whether a child has ADD, a comprehensive evaluation needs to be performed by professionals who are familiar with characteristics of the disorder.

STRESS
DISCOURAGEMENT
PHYSICAL ILLNESS
LEARNING DIFFICULTIES
FAMILY PROBLEMS

The process of evaluating whether a child has ADD usually involves a variety of professionals which can include the family physician, pediatrician, child and adolescent psychiatrist or psychologist, neurologist, family counselor and teacher. Psychiatric interview, psychological and educational testing, and/or a neurological examination can provide information leading to a proper diagnosis and treatment planning. An accurate diagnosis is necessary before proper treatment can begin. Complex cases in which the diagnosis is unclear or is complicated by other medical and psychiatric conditions should be seen by a physician.

Parents and teachers, being the primary sources of information about the child's ability to attend and focus at home and in school, play an integral part in the evaluation process.

3. What kinds of services and programs help children with ADD and their families?

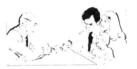

Help for the ADD child and the family is best provided through *multi-modal* treatment delivered by a team of professionals who look after the medical, emotional, behavioral, and educational needs of the child. Parents play an essential role as coordinators of services and programs designed to help their child. Such services and programs may include:

• Medication to help improve attention, and reduce impulsivity and hyperactivity, as well as to treat other emotional or adjustment problems which sometimes accompany ADD.

• Training parents to understand ADD and to be more effective behavior managers as well as advocates for their child.

• Counseling or training ADD children in methods of self-control, attention focusing, learning strategies, organizational skills, or social skill development.

• Psychotherapy to help the demoralized or even depressed ADD child.

• Other interventions at home and at school designed to enhance self-esteem and foster acceptance, approval, and a sense of belonging.

4. What medications are prescribed for ADD children?

Medications can dramatically improve attention span and reduce hyperactive and impulsive behavior. Psychostimulants have been used to treat attentional deficits in children since the 1940's. Antidepressants, while used less frequently to treat ADD, have been shown to be quite effective for the management of this disorder in some children.

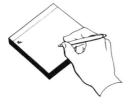

5. How do psychostimulants such as Dexedrine (dextroamphetamine), Ritalin (methylphenidate) and Cylert (pemoline) help?

Seventy to eighty per cent of ADD children respond in a positive manner to psychostimulant medication. Exactly how these medicines work is not known. However, benefits for children can be quite significant and are most apparent when concentration is required. In classroom settings, on-task behavior and completion of assigned tasks is increased, socialization with peers and teacher is improved, and disruptive behaviors (talking out, demanding attention, getting out of seat, noncompliance with requests, breaking rules) are reduced.

The specific dose of medicine must be determined for each child. Generally, the higher the dose, the greater the effect and side effects. To ensure proper dosage, regular monitoring at different levels should be done. Since there are no clear guidelines as to how long a child should take medication, periodic trials off medication should be done to determine continued need. Behavioral rating scales, testing on continuous performance tasks, and the child's self-reports provide helpful, but not infallible measures of progress.

Despite myths to the contrary, a positive response to stimulants is often found in adolescents with ADD, therefore, medication need not be discontinued as the child reaches adolescence if it is still needed.

6. What are common side effects of psychostimulant medications?

Reduction in appetite, loss of weight, and problems in falling asleep are the most common adverse effects. Children treated

with stimulants may become irritable and more sensitive to criticism or rejection. Sadness and a tendency to cry are occasionally seen.

The unmasking or worsening of a tic disorder is an infrequent effect of stimulants. In some cases this involves Tourette's Disorder. Generally, except in Tourette's, the tics decrease or disappear with the discontinuation of the stimulant. Caution must be employed in medicating adolescents with stimulants if there are coexisting disorders, e.g. depression, substance abuse, conduct, tic or mood disorders. Likewise, caution should be employed when a family history of a tic disorder exists.

Some side effects, e.g. decreased spontaneity, are felt to be dose-related and can be alleviated by reduction of dosage or switching to another stimulant. Similarly, slowing of height and weight gain of children on stimulants has been documented, with a return to normal for both occurring upon discontinuation of the medication. Other less common side effects have been described but they may occur as frequently with a placebo as with active medication. Pemoline may cause impaired liver functioning in 3% of children, and this may not be completely reversed when this medication is discontinued.

Over-medication has been reported to cause impairment in cognitive functioning and alertness. Some children on higher doses of stimulants will experience what has been described as a "rebound" effect, consisting of changes in mood, irritability and increases of the symptoms associated with their disorder. This occurs with variable degrees of severity during the late afternoon or evening, when the level of medicine in the blood falls. Thus, an additional low dose of medicine in the late afternoon or a decrease of the noontime dose might be required.

7. When are tricyclic antidepressants such as Tofranil (imipramine), Norpramin (desipramine) and Elavil (amytriptyline) used to treat ADD children?

This group of medications is generally considered when contraindications to stimulants exist, when stimulants have not been effective or have resulted in unacceptable side effects, or when the antidepressant property is more critical to treatment than the decrease of inattentiveness. They are used much less frequently than the stimulants, seem to have a different mechanism of action, and may be somewhat less effective than the psychostimulants in treating ADD. Long-term use of the tricyclics has not been well studied. Children with ADD who are also experiencing anxiety or depression may do best with an initial trial of a tricyclic antidepressant followed, if needed, with a stimulant for the more classic ADD symptoms.

8. What are the side effects of tricyclic antidepressant medications?

Side effects include constipation and dry mouth. Symptomatic treatment with stool softeners and sugar free gum or candy are usually effective in alleviating the discomfort. Confusion, elevated blood pressure, possible precipitation of manic-like behavior and inducement of seizures are uncommon side effects. The latter three occur in vulnerable individuals who can generally be identified during the assessment phase.

9. What about ADD children who do not respond well to medication?

Some ADD children or adolescents will not respond satisfactorily to either the psychostimulant or tricyclic antidepressant medications. Non-responders may have severe symptoms of ADD, may have other problems in addition to ADD, or may not be able to tolerate certain medications due to adverse side effects as noted above. In such cases consultation with a child and adolescent psychiatrist may be helpful.

10. How often should medications be dispensed at school to an ADD child?

Since the duration for effective action for Ritalin and Dexedrine, the most commonly used psychostimulants, is only about four hours, a second dose during school is often required. Taking a second dose of medication at noon-time enables the ADD child to focus attention effectively, utilize appropriate school behavior and maintain academic productivity. However, the noontime dose can sometimes be eliminated for children whose afternoon academic schedule does not require high levels of attentiveness. Some psychostimulants, i.e. SR Ritalin (sustained release form) and Cylert, work for longer periods of time (eight to ten hours) and may help avoid the need for a noon-time dose. Antidepressant medications used to treat ADD are usually taken in the morning, afternoon hours after school, or in the evening.

In many cases the physician may recommend that medication be continued at non-school times such as weekday afternoons, weekends or school vacations. During such non-school times lower doses of medication than those taken for school may be sufficient. It is important to remember that ADD is more than a school problem — it is a problem which often interferes in the learning of constructive social, peer, and sports activities.

11. How should medication be dispensed at school?

Most important, regardless of who dispenses medication, since an ADD child may already feel "different" from others, care should be taken to provide discreet reminders to the child when it is time to take medication. It is quite important that school personnel treat the administration of medication in a sensitive manner, thereby safeguarding the privacy of the child or adolescent and avoiding any unnecessary embarrassment. Success in doing this will increase the student's compliance in taking medication.

The location for dispensing medication at school may vary depending upon the school's resources. In those schools with a full-time nurse, the infirmary would be the first choice. In those schools in which a nurse is not always available, other properly trained school personnel may take the responsibility of supervising and dispensing medication.

12. How should the effectiveness of medication and other treatments for the ADD child be monitored?

Important information needed to judge the effectiveness of medication usually comes from reports by the child's parents and teachers and should include information about the child's behavior and attentiveness, academic performance, social and emotional adjustment and any medication side-effects.

Reporting from these sources may be informal through telephone, or more objective via the completion of scales designed for this purpose.

The commonly used teacher rating scales are:
- Conners Teacher Rating Scales
- ADD-H Comprehensive Teacher Rating Scale
- Child Behavior Checklist
- ADHD Rating Scale
- Child Attention Problems (CAP) Rating Scale
- School Situations Questionnaire

Academic performance should be monitored by comparing classroom grades prior to and after treatment.

It is important to monitor changes in peer relationships, family functioning, social skills, a capacity to enjoy leisure time, and self-esteem.

The parents, school nurse or other school personnel responsible for dispensing or overseeing the medication trial should have regular contact by phone with the prescribing physician. Physician office visits of sufficient frequency to monitor treatment are critical in the overall care of children with ADD.

13. What is the role of the teacher in the care of children with ADD?

Teaching an ADD child can test the limits of any educator's time and patience. As any parent of an ADD child will tell you, being on the front lines helping these children to manage on a daily basis can be both challenging and exhausting. It helps if teachers know what to expect and if they receive in-service training on how to teach

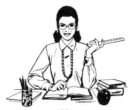

and manage ADD students in their classroom.

Here are some ideas that teachers told us have helped:
- Build upon the child's strengths by offering a great deal of encouragement and praise for the child's efforts, no matter how small.
- Learn to use behavior modification programs that motivate students to focus attention, behave better, and complete work.
- Talk with the child's parents and find helpful strategies that have worked with the child in the past.
- If the child is taking medication, communicate frequently with the physician (and parents) so that proper adjustments can be made with respect to type or dose of medication. Behavior rating scales are good for this purpose.
- Modify the classroom structure to accommodate the child's span of attention, i.e. shorter assignments, preferential seating in the classroom, appealing curriculum material, animated presentation of lessons, and frequent positive reinforcement.
- Determine whether the child can be helped through special educational resources within the school.
- Consult with other school personnel such as the guidance counselor, school psychologist, or school nurse to get their ideas as well.

14. What are common myths associated with ADD medications?

Myth: Medication should be stopped when a child reaches teen years.

Fact: Research clearly shows that there is continued benefit to medication for those teens who meet criteria for diagnosis of ADD.

Myth: Children build up a tolerance to medication.

Fact: Although the dose of medication may need adjusting from time to time there is no evidence that children build up a tolerance to medication.

Myth: Taking medication for ADD leads to greater likelihood of later drug addiction.

Fact: There is no evidence to indicate that ADD medication leads to an increased likelihood of later drug addiction.

Myth: Positive response to medication is confirmation of a diagnosis of ADD.

Fact: The fact that a child shows improvement of attention span or a reduction of activity while taking ADD medication does not substantiate the diagnosis of ADD. Even some normal children will show a marked improvement in attentiveness when they take ADD medications.

Myth: Medication stunts growth.

Fact: ADD medications may cause an initial and mild slowing of growth, but over time the growth suppression effect is minimal if non-existent in most cases.

Myth: Taking ADD medications as a child makes you more reliant on drugs as an adult.

Fact: There is no evidence of increased medication taking when medicated ADD children become adults, nor is there evidence that ADD children become addicted to their medications.

Myth: ADD children who take medication attribute their success only to medication.

Fact: When self-esteem is encouraged, a child taking medication attributes his success not only to the medication but to himself as well.

Summary of Important Points

1. ADD children make up 3-5% of the population, but many children who have trouble paying attention may have problems other than ADD. A thorough evaluation can help determine whether attentional deficits are due to ADD or to other conditions.

2. Once identified, ADD children are best treated with a *multi-modal* approach. Best results are obtained when behavioral management programs, educational interventions, parent training, counseling, and medication, when needed, are used together to help the ADD child. Parents of children and adolescents with ADD play the key role of coordinating these services.

3. Each ADD child responds in his or her own unique way to medication depending upon the child's physical make-up, severity of ADD symptoms, and other possible problems accompanying the ADD. Responses to medication need to be monitored and reported to the child's physician.

4. Teachers play an essential role in helping the ADD child feel comfortable within the classroom procedures and work demands, sensitivity to self-esteem issues, and frequent parent-teacher contact can help a great deal.

5. ADD may be a life-long disorder requiring life-long assistance. Families, and the children themselves, need our continued support and understanding.

6. Successful treatment of the medical aspects of ADD is dependent upon ongoing collaboration between the prescribing physician, teacher, therapist and parents.

APPENDIX M

HYPERACTIVITY AND FOOD ADDITIVES[6]

National Advisory Committee on Hyperkinesis and
Food Additives
Nutrition Foundation, New York, New York, October, 1980

"It is our opinion that the studies already completed provide sufficient evidence to refute the claim that artificial food coloring, artificial flavorings and salicylates produce hyperactivity and/or learning disability .... Since the food additive-free diet has no harmful effects, and since the non-specific (Placebo) effects of this dietary treatment are frequently very beneficial to families, we see no reason to discourage those families who wish to pursue this type of treatment as long as they continue to follow other therapy that is helpful. If the family asks, however, for the clinician's advice, he or she must cope with the ethical issues involved in recommending a treatment for its placebo effect while the family believes that the treatment is based upon scientific evidence."

Quote from Sydney S. Gellis, M.D.:   "The members of this committee are academicians of solid worth and standing."

APPENDIX N

POSITION STATEMENT*
American Academy of Allergy and Immunology

CANDIDIASIS HYPERSENSITIVITY SYNDROME

Candida Albicans is a type of germ known as a yeast or fungus. It is normally present on the mucous membranes of most people. However, identifying Candida on the membranes or in secretions does not indicate disease.

People who lack normal body defenses, people with immune deficiency diseases, and some people whose normal germ balance has been affected by antibiotic therapy may have an overgrowth of Candida. This imbalance usually causes no symptoms and eventually corrects itself without treatment, but it may cause some discomfort. For example, vaginal Candida overgrowth can cause itching and discharge. These occasional problems are unpleasant but are not dangerous.

Some individuals have publicized the unproven theory that Candida infection often causes serious symptoms and constitutes a major health problem for many people. They claim that Candida can cause a variety of symptoms including fatigue, depression, inability to concentrate, hyperactivity, headaches, skin rashes, digestive pains and bloating, bleeding problems, and reproductive organ problems. Although such general symptoms and signs can occur in many well-defined diseases, advocates of the Candida *connection* always relate these problems to the so-called "Candida Syndrome."

*Paraphrased by the Subcommittee for Public Information on Acceptable Medical Practice.[19]

It is important to know that all of these symptoms and their *connection* with yeast are unproven. Many people have experienced one or more of these problems at some time, so many are attracted to the claim that Candida is responsible. However, there is neither clinical nor laboratory proof that Candida causes any of the wide range of symptoms mentioned above.

In addition, there is no proof that the large number of remedies for "Candida Syndrome" do any good. These remedies include exercise, mental health counseling, avoidance of chemical pollutants, special diets that restrict sugars, dyes and preservatives, yeast-free diets, nutritional supplements and use of antifungal medications. Actually, there is a risk that long-term use of antifungal medications may cause more dangerous strains of germs to grow in the body. It is quite possible that those who try these remedies will suffer restriction of lifestyle for no proven benefit.

If you hear or read about the "Candida Syndrome" and you feel that your own symptoms fit the description, remember that anyone might have these problems sometime and that they may develop from a wide variety of causes. Blaming Candida sounds easy, but there is no scientific proof that Candida can cause such a wide spectrum of unrelated disease symptoms. Objective laboratory tests have not confirmed Candida as the cause of symptoms in people who believe they have the so-called "Candida Syndrome."

Reprinted with permission of American Academy of Allergy and Immunology, Journal of Allergy and Clinical Immunology, August, 1986.

APPENDIX O

HUGGING

Hugs are not only nice; they're needed. Hugs can relieve pain and depressions, make the healthy healthier, the happy happier, and the most secure among us even more so.

Hugging feels good, overcomes fear, eases tension, provides stretching exercise if you're short, and stooping exercise if you're tall.

Hugging does not upset the environment, saves heat and requires no special equipment. It makes happy days happier and impossible days possible.

Author Unknown

Reprinted with permission of Kathy Tobin, <u>Tomahawk Wisconsin Leader</u>, 1988.

APPENDIX P

National Support Groups

Attention Deficit Disorders Association (ADDA)
P. O. Box 488
West Newbury, MA 01985 (800) 487-2282

Children with Attention Deficit Disorders (CHADD)
499 N.W. 70th Avenue, Suite 308
Plantation, FL 33317 (305) 587-3700

Learning Disabilities Association of America (LDA)
4156 Library Road
Pittsburgh, PA 15234 (412) 341-1515

Tourette Syndrome Association (TSA)
42-40 Bell Boulevard
Bayside, NY 11361 (718) 224-2999

GLOSSARY

Behavior pill—What Ritalin is not. [Page 65]

Biologic morality—What Dr. George Still probably meant when, in 1902, he spoke of moral control beyond parental influence. [Page 3]

Blurt ratio—A specific test for ADD employed by first grade teachers. [Page 30]

Boring—The commonest utterance of a child with ADD. [Page 39]

Datsun child—The hyperactive child without ADD - he is driven. [Page 21]

Flypaper attention—Overfocused attention which persons with ADD may demonstrate at times - they get stuck. [Page 20]

Himalaya profile—Produced by connecting the dots on an ADD child's achievement test score sheet. [Page 57]

How comes?—Questions to be avoided when dealing with a child with ADD. [Page 96]

Hug therapy—Beneficial to all - a necessity for the child with ADD. [Page 103]

Hypoaroused—What *Jumpin' Johnnie* does not appear to be but maybe he is. [Page 26]

Lethal cluster—The academic nemesis of children with ADD and LD. [Page 102]

Maternal hormone—Guilt. [Page 11]

Mel's malevolence—Success deprivation - bad stuff. [Page 94]

Mimics—ADD look-alikes but aren't ADD. [Page 15]

Sound sleeper—The person with ADD who makes sounds while he sleeps - night terrors are common. [Page 39]

Squeaky wheel—Boys with ADD are more likely to get diagnostic grease than their less boisterous female counterparts. [Page 9]

Squirm count—Valuable tests of task irrelevant physical activity. [Page 29]

Telephone magnet—Unscrew the plastic speaker cover and you will find it—it attracts verbal utterances from the ADD child as soon as his mother initiates a phone conversation. [Page 31]

Wide angle lens—Refers to the ability of the child with ADD to take it all in all at one time. [Page 36]

Zombie—Not created by reasonable Ritalin dosage. [Page 75]

FOOTNOTES

1. Fleishman, Cindy.   Quote from my daughter, a regular classroom teacher who applies special education skills to her work.

2. American Psychiatric Association (1980). *Diagnostic and Statistical Manual of Mental Disorders (Third Edition)*. Washington, D.C.: Author.

3. American Psychiatric Association (1987). *Diagnostic and Statistical Manual of Mental Disorders (Third edition-revised-DSM-III-R)*. Washington, D.C.: Author.

4. Zametkin, Alan J., et al. (1990). Cerebral Glucose Metabolism in Adults with Hyperactivity of Childhood Onset.   *New England Journal of Medicine, 323*(20):1361-66.

5. Comings, David E. et al. (1991). The Dopamine D2 Receptor Locus as a Modifying Gene in Neuropsychiatric Disorders. *Journal of the American Medical Association, 266*:1793-1807.

6. National Advisory Committee on Hyperkinesis and Food Additives (1980). "Hyperactivity and Food Additives," Nutrition Foundation, New York.

7. Dismukes, William E., et al. (1990). A randomized double-blind trial of nystatin therapy for the Candidiasis Hypersensitivity Syndrome. *The New England Journal of Medicine, 323*(25).

8. Bennett, John E. (1990). Searching for the yeast connection. *The New England Journal of Medicine, 323*(25).

9. Conners, C. Keith. (1989). *Feeding the Brain*. New York: Plenum Press.

10. Lahey, Benjamin. (1991). "Attention Deficit Disorder Without Hyperactivity." Address, Third Annual CH.A.D.D. Conference, Washington. D.C., September 20.

11. Barkley, Russell, A. (1990). *Attention Deficit Hyperactivity Disorder: A Handbook for Diagnosis and Treatment.* New York: Guilford Press.

12. Gordon, Michael. (1991). *Jumpin' Johnnie Get Back to Work. A Child's Guide to ADHD/Hyperactivity.* De Witt, NY: GSI Publications.

13. Capsela.® A registered trademark of Mitsubishi Pencil Co. under license by Play-Jour International, Tokyo. Distributed in the United States by Sanyei-America Corp., Secaucus, NJ.

14. Landy, Sarah and Peters, Ray DeV. (1990). Identifying and treating aggressive preschoolers. *Infants and Young Children,* 3(2):24-38.

15. Barkley, R.A., DuPaul, E.J., and McMurry, M.B. (1991). Attention deficit disorder with and without hyperactivity: Clinical response to methylphenidate. *Pediatrics, 87:*519-531.

16. Copeland, E. D. (1991). *Medications for Attention Disorders (ADHD/ADD) and Related Medical Problems.* Atlanta: SPI Press.

17. "The Responsibility of the School Under Federal Law", in Copeland, E. D. (1991), *Medications for Attention Disorders (ADHD/ADD) and Related Medical Problems.* Atlanta: SPI Press.

18. Golden, G.S. (1988). The relationship between stimulant medication and tics. *Pediatric Annals, 17(6):*405-408.

19. American Academy of Allergy and Immunology (1986). "Position statement: Candidiasis hypersensitivity syndrome." *Journal of Allergy and Immunology,* August: 269-277.